Management of Temporomandibular Joint Degenerative Diseases:

Biologic Basis and Treatment Outcome

Edited by

■ B. Stegenga
■ L.G.M. de Bont

Birkhäuser Verlag
Basel · Boston · Berlin

Editors:

Boudewijn Stegenga, DDS, PhD
Department of Oral and Maxillofacial Surgery
University Hospital Groningen
P. O. Box 30.001
9700 RB Groningen
The Netherlands

Lambert G. M. de Bont, DDS, PhD
Professor and Chairman
Department of Oral and Maxillofacial Surgery
University Hospital Groningen
P. O. Box 30.001
9700 RB Groningen
The Netherlands

A CIP catalogue record for this book is available from the Library of Congress, Washington, D.C., USA

Deutsche Bibliothek Cataloging-in-Publication Data

Management of temporomandibular joint degenerative diseases
: biologic basis and treatment outcome / ed. by B. Stegenga ;
L. G. M. de Bont. - Basel ; Boston ; Berlin : Birkhäuser, 1996
ISBN-13: 978-3-0348-9859-1   e-ISBN-13: 978-3-0348-8992-6
DOI: 10.1007/978-3-0348-8992-6
NE: Stegenga, Boudewijn [Hrsg.]

9 8 7 6 5 4 3 2 1

This book is dedicated to Professor Geert Boering

Contents

Introduction

Treatment planning

Surgical procedures: biologic basis and treatment outcome

Post-operative care and treatment failure

Synthesis

Foreword

It is fashionable in professional circles to deplore the difficulty of intellectual discourse between "academicians" – men of letters, researchers, rationalists – and "practitioners" – surgeons, radiologists, physical therapists. How beneficial it would be if educated non-academicians could speak intelligently about *t*-tests and chi-square tests and men of academia could appreciate the travail, spirit, and needs of a busy office and practice!

Even this suspected gap between "two cultures" came very near together in the wonderful town of Groningen (The Netherlands) as wise men from both practice and scholarship gathered to talk about the unfathomables of the temporomandibular joint. There were keen discussions about the intense biological changes which occur about the complex temporomandibular joint after excessive use or injury. These papers were followed by talks outlining the experiences of those involved in the imaging and non-surgical and surgical management of patients who were enduring such changes. The pitch and interchange of opinions and evidence as to why a disc or its position could effect little or profound disturbance of the temporomandibular apparatus were enlightening to each who listened – and thought. And even more sobering was to hear the report of a well-documented, multiple decades long study of a large number of patients with osteoarthrosis and internal derangement which defined a natural course and eventual end of the disease. With this understanding, one is now faced with the obvious question of how much treatment patients with osteoarthrosis really require.

There was infinitely more to the conference than agonizing with osteoarthrosis and internal derangements. So much has been said and now written about the interrelation of the two that special attention was given to discussion of that correlation. But ample time was provided for talk involving treatment planning, occlusion, measurement of treatment outcomes, imaging, arthroscopy, arthrocentesis, open surgery, rehabilitation, physical therapy, ankylosis following previous surgery, and management of non-successful treatment – all related to the joint under scrutiny, the temporomandibular joint. There was balance to the Conference and there were enough areas of disagreement concerning diagnosis and treatment that everyone in attendance was provoked in due time to have his objective view heard.

Groningen was a natural venue for this important conference and the hearing of so many distinguished workers in the ideology of temporomandibular disorders and those involved in creative care of these patients. For years the University Hospital Groningen has maintained probably the most outstanding academic program in oral and maxillofacial surgery in the world with a primary concentration in basic temporomandibular joint investigations. The flow of PhD theses and research reports relative to temporomandibular joint concerns from this institution have spawned hundreds of scientific articles about this joint around the world. The eminent speakers attracted to Groningen for this conference have proven to be true innovators regarding temporomandibular joint study and each in all likelihood has been influenced by the work which has come from this ancient and delightful city. These speakers reflect individuals driven by interest in a problem and a need to refine care, dominate their own idea, and create a predictable treatment. Even though much understanding was gained from the many papers and the innovative treatment of a common problem, it is clear that not all answers for a unified approach to temporomandibular joint care have yet been provided. Steffens correctly stated: "Nothing is done. Everything in the world remains to be done or done over." But this collection of chapters based on the conference will be of immense value to everyone working at both the academic and practice levels of temporomandibular joint matters. Even so, it is sensible to heed T.S. Eliot's thoughtful words:

> "Between the idea
> And the reality
> Between the motion
> And the act
> Falls the Shadow ..."

We are still in a shadow under which we need to further clarify the truths regarding the origin and course of temporomandibular joint ailments and to develop a prudent course in the management of them. The conference in Groningen has launched us in a good direction with an improved appreciation of the need for further study of temporomandibular afflictions and their care.

Robert V. Walker
Professor and Past Chairman
Diplomate, American Board of Oral and Maxillofacial Surgeons
The University of Texas Southwestern Medical Center
Division of Oral and Maxillofacial Surgery
Dallas, Texas
USA

Contributors

Quentin N. Anderson, HCMC Department of Medical Imaging, University of Minnesota, Minneapolis, Minnesota 55415-1829, USA

Lambert G. M. de Bont, Department of Oral and Maxillofacial Surgery, University Hospital Groningen, 9700 RB Groningen, The Netherlands

Pieter U. Dijkstra, Department of Oral and Maxillofacial Surgery, Division of Physical Therapy, Department of Rehabilitation, University Hospital Groningen, 9700 RB Groningen, The Netherlands

M. Franklin Dolwick, Oral and Maxillofacial Surgery, University of Florida College of Dentistry, Gainesville, Florida 32610, USA

John F. Helfrick, Department of Oral and Maxillofacial Surgery, University of Texas at Houston, Health Science Center, Dental Branch, Houston, Texas 77030, USA

Anders B. Holmlund, Department of Oral and Maxillofacial Surgery, School of Dentistry, Karolinska Institute, 14104 Huddinge, Sweden

Bart van der Kuijl, Department of Oral and Maxillofacial Surgery, University Hospital Groningen, 9700 RB Groningen, The Netherlands

Robert B. MacIntosh, Department of Dentistry and Oral and Maxillofacial Surgery, Sinai Hospital of Detroit, Detroit, Michigan 48025, USA

William L. McCarty, Oral and Maxillofacial Surgery, Baptist Medical Center, Montgomery, Alabama 36198, USA

Samuel J. McKenna, Department of Oral and Maxillofacial Surgery, Vanderbilt University School of Medicine, Nashville, Tennessee 37232, USA

Ralph G. Merrill, Department of Oral and Maxillofacial Surgery, School of Dentistry, Oregon Health Sciences University, Portland, Oregon 97201-3097, USA

Ken-Ichiro Murakami, Department of Oral and Maxillofacial Surgery, Faculty of Medicine, Kyoto University Hospital, Kyoto, Japan

Dorrit W. Nitzan, Department of Oral and Maxillofacial Surgery, Faculty of Dental Medicine, The Hebrew University, Hadassah School of Dental Medicine, 91120 Jerusalem, Israel

Jeffrey P. Okeson, Orofacial Pain Center, University of Kentucky College of Dentistry, Lexington, Kentucky 40536-0084, USA

Rudolf H. Reich, Department of Oral and Maxillofacial Surgery, Rheinische Friedrich-Wilhelms University, D-53111 Bonn, Germany

Doran E. Ryan, Department of Oral and Maxillofacial Surgery, Medical College of Wisconsin, Milwaukee, Wisconsin 53226, USA

Robert D. Schwartz, Department of Oral and Maxillofacial Surgery, University of Illinois and Northwestern University, Chicago, Illinois 60602, USA

Natsuki Segami, Department of Oral and Maxillofacial Surgery, Faculty of Medicine, Kyoto University Hospital, Kyoto, Japan

Boudewijn Stegenga, Department of Oral and Maxillofacial Surgery, University Hospital Groningen, 9700 RB Groningen, The Netherlands

D. Bram Tuinzing, Department of Oral and Maxillofacial Surgery/Oral Pathology, University Hospital VU/ACTA, 1007 MB Amsterdam, The Netherlands

Preface

This text features the biologic basis for the clinical management of complex temporomandibular joint diseases. The chapters are based on the International TMJ Conference on the Management of Temporomandibular Joint Degenerative Diseases, held in Groningen, The Netherlands, in honor of Prof. Dr. Geert Boering.

The primary aim of this text is to present differing points of view with regard to the pathophysiology, diagnosis, and management of temporomandibular joint degenerative diseases. The considerable number of contributors reflects the diversity of approaches to the problems facing us. Despite this diversity, the book intends to provide a useful basis for decision-making in the management of temporomandibular joint degenerative disorders.

The text is subdivided into four sections. The first two sections focus on treatment planning, and serve as a basis for the other sections. Treatment planning should initially be based on clinical presentation, and should take into account any underlying pathology (Drs. de Bont, Stegenga, Dolwick). Furthermore, it is important to provide adequate non-surgical management (Dr. Okeson) as well as to specify clearly the criteria for surgical management of these disorders (Dr. Reich). This is essential, because the disorder may not be at a stage that requires surgical treatment. Moreover, several temporomandibular disorders never require surgical management, while other aspects related to the patient's status (e.g., orthognathic considerations) may influence the treatment planning process (Dr. Tuinzing). Both clinically and scientifically, outcome criteria should be clearly defined prior to the therapy (Dr. Holmlund). Finally, appropriate imaging procedures remain important in planning treatment for temporomandibular disorders, especially when it concerns surgical management (Drs. van der Kuijl, Anderson, and Murakami).

In the third section, the biologic basis and outcome of several surgical procedures is discussed. The presentations at the International TMJ Conference were given by leading authorities with considerable clinical experience in arthrocentesis and arthroscopic procedures (Drs. Nitzan, Schwartz, McCain, and Koslin), condylotomy (Dr. McKenna), and open joint procedures (Drs. Ryan, and Piper). We are grateful that most of these contributions could be included in this text.

The fourth section focuses on post-operative care and rehabilitation (Drs. McCarty and Dijkstra), and on management of treatment failure (Drs. MacIntosh and Merrill).

At the conclusion of the conference, seven controversial statements were discussed by an expert panel and conference participants. The discussion was chaired by Dr. John F. Helfrick (USA), and the panel consisted of Drs. Alastair Goss (Australia), Lars Eriksson (Sweden), and Jeffrey Okeson (USA).

We are especially grateful to those who contributed to the conference and to this book. We very much appreciate the continuing stimulating support of the staff of Birkhäuser Publishing Ltd., Basel, Switzerland.

The text will be of interest to all who are involved in the management of temporomandibular joint degenerative diseases, be it from a clinical, biologic, or scientific background.

Boudewijn Stegenga
Lambert G.M. de Bont

Introduction

Management of Temporomandibular
Joint Degenerative Diseases
ed. by B. Stegenga & L.G.M. de Bont
© 1996 Birkhäuser Verlag Basel/Switzerland

Temporomandibular joint degenerative diseases: pathogenesis

Lambert G.M. de Bont

Department of Oral and Maxillofacial Surgery, University Hospital Groningen, 9700 RB Groningen, The Netherlands

Summary: The pathology of temporomandibular joint osteoarthrosis involves synovial joint pathology and connective tissue diseases. It is becoming increasingly obvious that enzymatic pathways, in addition to mechanical factors, are involved in cartilage matrix degradation. In order to establish an effective regimen of therapy, it is important to understand how matrix degradation develops and what enzymes mediate this process. This chapter focuses on current knowledge with regard to the degenerative process occurring in temporomandibular joint osteoarthrosis.

Introduction

Temporomandibular joint disorders include non-inflammatory chondro-osteoarthropathies (e.g., osteoarthrosis and internal derangement), primary arthritides (e.g., rheumatoid arthritis, psoriatic arthritis), and secondary arthritides (e.g., osteoarthritis, crystal-induced arthropathies).[1] Osteoarthrosis is a slowly progressive, usually monoarticular disorder that is inherently non-inflammatory.[2,3] The disorder is characterized by progressive degradation of components of the extracellular matrix of articular cartilage.[4]

Research with regard to osteoarthrosis was initially confined to histopathologic and electron microscopic changes in human osteoarthrotic cartilage, but the last decade has focused on biochemical and metabolic changes. This change in perspective has influenced the definition of osteoarthrosis. Currently, osteoarthrosis is defined as resulting from an imbalance between predominantly chondrocyte-controlled anabolic and catabolic processes. It is characterized by progressive degradation of components of the extracellular matrix of articular cartilage, with secondary inflammatory components.[4] Many interacting enzymes and cytokines are involved in this cartilage degradation process, and undoubtedly more factors will be discovered in the future. Due to the limited availability of human cartilage, especially in the early stages of the disease, many data regarding these changes are derived from animal model studies and *in vitro* cartilage explant studies.

The relationship between osteoarthrosis and internal derangement of the temporomandibular joint is commonly emphasized in the literature. Although osteoarthrosis may develop without disc displacement, internal derangement is highly correlated with temporomandibular joint osteoarthrosis.[5]

The pathologic state in the temporomandibular joint appears to be comparable to that in other synovial joints.[6] Consequently, temporomandibular joint pathology is synovial joint pathology, and the terminology used should be synovial joint terminology.[7,8]

Normal physiology of synovial joints: structure, function, biochemistry, and metabolism

Articular cartilage, synovial membrane, and synovial fluid are the basic elements of a synovial joint. The temporomandibular joint obeys the same biologic laws as do other synovial joints in the body, despite the difference between this joint and most other synovial joints regarding the type of articular cartilage, i.e., fibrocartilage versus hyaline cartilage. Synovial fluid covers the articular surface, and its presence is essential for joint lubrication and nutrition. Nutrition of the articular cartilage cells occurs by diffusion of molecules from the synovial fluid. Intermittent pumping during dynamic loading generates micro-circulatory currents in the region of the cartilage cells, which facilitates the transport of the cellularly derived matrix vesicles and all other products from and towards the cells. Consequently, changes in the synovial membrane probably cause changes in the synovial fluid content and, therefore, changes in cartilage metabolism.

Articular cartilage is composed of chondrocytes and matrix. Chondrocytes are active cells. They produce the collagen and the proteoglycans of the matrix, and also glycoproteins and enzymes. The collagen fibrils in temporomandibular joint articular cartilage are organized in a three-dimensional network of layers and bundles.[9] The proteoglycans, which are complex molecules composed of a protein core and numerous glycosaminoglycan chains, are connected to a hyaluronic acid chain and in this way create proteoglycan aggregates. These macromolecules, which are hydrophilic and form a gel that tends to swell, are situated between the collagen fibrils of the articular cartilage. They occupy the interstitial spaces in the matrix and are intertwined throughout the collagen network. This collagen network counteracts the swelling pressure of the proteoglycan aggregates. The proteoglycans thus keep the collagen network under constant tension. During normal functioning, the external pressure from loading will be in equilibrium with the internal cartilage pressure, which accounts for the physical properties of the articular cartilage.[10]

Proteases, cytokines, growth factors, and arachidonic acid metabolites are involved in the biochemistry and metabolism of normal and osteoarthritic cartilage.[11] Proteases or proteolytic enzymes play an important role both in maintaining normal tissue turnover and in the degradation of extracellular matrix components of articular cartilage in the osteoarthrotic process. Proteases are capable of cleaving internal peptide bonds of proteins.[12] Normal articular cartilage contains large amounts of protease inhibitors, including tissue inhibitor of metalloproteases and plasminogen activator inhibitor. An imbalance between proteases and protease inhibitor levels has been postulated as a possible pathogenic pathway of osteoarthrosis.[13]

Cytokines and growth factors are soluble polypeptides, capable of regulating growth, differentiation, and metabolic activity of cells.[14,15] Generally, cytokines (e.g., interleukin-I to -XII, tumor necrosis factor, interferon) exert a catabolic effect in articular cartilage, whereas growth factors (e.g., insulin-like growth factor, transforming growth factor, and fibroblast growth factor) exert an anabolic effect. Cytokines induce protease production, which may result in proteoglycan depletion in cartilage, and consequently increase the rate of cartilage degradation and decrease the rate of proteoglycan synthesis and other matrix components.

Arachidonic acid metabolites are inflammatory mediators. In response to specific stimuli, arachidonic acid is released from cell membrane phospholipids. Subsequently, it is converted to several prostaglandins and tromboxanes by the cyclo-oxygenase pathway, and to several leukotrienes by the lipoxygenase pathway.[16] Arachidonic acid metabolites can be synthesized by synovial cells, mediated by cytokines. Prostaglandin E_2 is a major mediator of inflammation, and its synthesis is induced by interleukin-I.[17]

Degeneration of synovial joints

If a primary insult, whether (bio)mechanical, biochemical, inflammatory, or immunologic in character, disturbs the chondrocyte-controlled balance between synthesis and degradation of extracellular matrix components, cartilage degradation ensues. Initially, cartilage degradation will be counteracted by attempts at repair.[18]

In the early stage of osteoarthrosis, the increased synthesis of extracellular matrix components is exceeded by their degradation due to increased synthesis and activity of proteases, resulting in (initially focal) degradation and loss of articular cartilage. In early degenerative changes, swelling and softening of the articular cartilage (chondromalacia), resulting from an increased volume of the proteoglycanwater gel, is observed. This presumably results from localized breakdown of collagen fibrils within the matrix due to collagenolytic activity. Since no cartilage components other than collagen have tensile strength, collagen fibril fragmentation seems to be the most acceptable explanation for the increased hydration of the articular cartilage. In addition to increased water content and collagen fibril fragmentation, proteoglycan depletion and clustering of chondrocytes are observed in early stage osteoarthrosis. The cells proliferate and become very active, in an attempt to repair the lost matrix.[19] The ratio of metalloproteases and their inhibitors increases, resulting in more proteolytic activity. Once cartilage degradation has started, the breakdown products are released into the synovial fluid and phagocytosed by the synovial membrane, resulting in an inflammatory response.[20] Consequently, the synovial fluid composition as well as the synovial membrane changes.[21]

There are several hypotheses regarding cartilage degeneration. The primary insult may be mechanical, chemical, or inflammatory, all resulting in chondrocyte or synovial cell breakdown, a release of proteolytic enzymes, and finally matrix degradation. When cartilage degeneration continues, the tissue loses its integrity, resulting in blistering, fibrillation, horizontal splitting, adhesion formation, cartilage thinning, and responses in adjacent tissues.

Mechanical forces to which articular cartilage is normally exposed are insufficient to destroy the tissue directly. Direct mechanical damage may occur when the chemical integrity of the matrix has been compromised. Hypotheses regarding the pathogenesis of osteoarthrosis include the relationship between loading and cartilage degradation: both biomechanical failure of articular cartilage and chondrocyte injury or failing chondrocyte response may result in degenerative changes. These degenerative changes are the result of an imbalance between the anabolic and catabolic activities of the articular cartilage or an imbalance between repair and degradation processes within the tissue. A modern definition of osteoarthrosis includes this mechanism:[14] osteoarthrosis is a disruption of a steadystate balance in a complex of interacting degradative and repair processes in cartilage, bone, and synovium with secondary inflammatory components.

The etiopathogenesis of osteoarthrosis probably involves a biochemically induced cascade of events in cartilage breakdown.[22] Extensive *in vitro* studies with cartilage explant cultures have demonstrated the significant role of degradative enzymes in cartilage breakdown. Animal models with artificially induced osteoarthrosis have shown the same mechanisms.

Cartilage breakdown and cartilage repair are dual processes which are continuously present. Breakdown is caused by collagenolytic and proteolytic enzymes; repair is expressed by chondrocyte proliferation and increased synthesis of collagen and proteoglycans. In both processes, and therefore in the control of homeostasis, chondrocytes appear to have a key function.

The cell is surrounded by numerous peptide factors which modulate the growth and differentiation of cartilage cells. There is increasing evidence that any one of these factors may influence the production and biological effects of other factors, yielding a very complex interactive system. The involved peptide factors and proteases are nowadays classified as cytokines, growth factors, metalloproteases, and tissue inhibitor of metalloproteases. All seem to play a critical role in the regulation of cartilage degradation and repair during normal and pathological turnover of the cartilage matrix.[11,22] There are several hypotheses about the role of cytokines, growth factors, metalloproteases, and tissue inhibitors of metalloproteases in the etiopathogenesis of osteoarthrosis. A general feature in these hypotheses is an imbalance between the amount of metalloproteases and their tissue inhibitors, corresponding to a relative deficit of inhibitors.

Stromelysin, collagenase, and gelatinase are the major metalloproteases. Their synthesis and secretion by the chondrocytes may be influenced by the presence of interleukin-I. This is one of the major cytokines which is produced by the synovial lining cells and other cells (e.g., chondrocytes). Thus, the action of interleukin-I results in a chondrocyte-mediated depletion of matrix proteoglycans, in addition to inadequate repair of the damaged matrix. In addition, interleukin-I increases the synthesis of proteases by the synovial lining cells in the osteoarthrotic joint. Synovial metalloprotease production seems to correlate with the severity of synovial inflammation, and the severity of synovial inflammation with the level of interleukin-I in the synovial fluid.

The intermediate stage of osteoarthrosis is characterized biochemically by a failing synthesis of extracellular matrix components, whereas the synthesis of proteases remains increased, mediated by the network of interacting cytokines.

The late stage of osteoarthrosis may be characterized biochemically by a continued increased synthesis of proteases, or by a decreased synthesis of proteases in the case of residual osteoarthrosis. The content of several extracellular matrix components is further reduced in this stage.

Osteoarthrosis of the temporomandibular joint

Osteoarthrosis affects not only the articular cartilage but also the subchondral bone, the synovial lining cells, the synovial fluid, and the capsular ligaments.[23] Osteoarthritis includes an inflammatory component caused by waste products and inflammatory mediators (i.e., osteoarthritis is an osteoarthrosis with synovitis).

In the "temporomandibular joint osteoarthrosis concept", different conditions of the articular cartilage are described, i.e., from normal variation to initial degenerative changes, from initial degenerative changes to advanced changes, and finally to destroyed cartilage.[24] Throughout life, the articular cartilage and underlying bone display shifting equilibria between changes in form and function by tissue remodeling, just as all other joints do. The tissues adapt to applied stresses. When loading is beyond the limits of the system, compensatory responses may lead to new steady states.

Increased loading may stimulate remodeling, involving increased synthesis of proteoglycans and collagen fibrils. Overloading may disturb the equilibrium between form and function and give rise to tissue breakdown. Only severe overloading will cause irreversible changes and damage. Remodeling, both progressive and regressive, takes place continuously. When regressive remodeling dominates, shortening of the mandibular ascending ramus eventually results. Thus, there seems to be a distinct relationship between the adaptive capacity of articular cartilage, joint loading, and degenerative cartilage breakdown.

Chondromalacia is a term used rather loosely by the medical profession to describe a clinically distinctive post-traumatic softening of the articular cartilage of the patella in young persons. This term is now also currently applied to the temporomandibular joint. The anatomic lesions are microscopically indistinguishable from those of early osteoarthrosis.[25] Osteoarthrosis starts focally in a joint. Only when it is present to a certain degree does it become clinically manifest. Light microscopic characteristics of osteoarthrotic cartilage include fibrillation, splitting, thinning, clustering of chondrocytes, and a very irregular interface between subchondral bone and calcified cartilage. In the temporomandibular joint, the articular zone, i.e., the cartilage layer at the articular surface, frequently seems unaffected, while degenerative changes such as horizontal splitting, fibrosis of the bone marrow, and clustering of chondrocytes are clearly present in the deeper layers of the tissue.[25] None of these phenomena are detectable during arthroscopic inspection or during open-joint surgery.

Splitting of the articular cartilage at the interface between calcified and uncalcified cartilage is basically the process that causes osteochondritis dissecans. Some magnetic resonance imaging studies suggest that osteochondritis dissecans is a real clinical entity.[26]

Radiographically detectable degenerative changes of the temporomandibular joint include lipping caused by osteophyte formation, sclerosis, surface erosions, subchondral cysts, and deformation. Most of these changes are visible during, but not curable by, surgical procedures.

Relationship between osteoarthrosis and internal derangement

Cartilage breakdown in osteoarthrosis affects the sliding properties of the joint surfaces. Deterioration of the synovial fluid in osteoarthrosis gives rise to friction and adhesive wear. Both impair the movement of the disc and may cause disc hesitation. This may induce joint stiffness and repetitive stretching of the disc attachments. The attachments may gradually elongate to an extent that permits disc displacement. This sequence of events explains the relationship between osteoarthrosis and internal derangements of the temporomandibular joint.[23]

Based on these assumptions, when classifying temporomandibular arthropathies, osteoarthrosis with and without disc displacement should be distinguished.[27] Secondary osteoarthrosis is the result of other joint disorders, e.g., rheumatoid arthritis, avascular necrosis, and osteochondritis dissecans.

Although disc displacement is a real clinical entity, the position and form of a physiologically functioning disc have certain variations.[28] A twelve o'clock position of the posterior band of the disc is no longer a standard of normal, since asymptomatic normal subjects show disc malposition and deformity in a significant portion of the studied population. This suggests that a large percentage of patients have a different basis for their intracapsular symptoms than only disc displacement. Thus, whether disc displacement is a cause or a sign of temporomandibular joint osteoarthrosis remains unclear.

Discussion

Because of its relative isolation from factors normally carried by the circulation, due to the absence of capillaries, and the abundance of proteoglycans which limit the diffusion of these factors, articular cartilage was once thought of as an inert tissue[18]. Currently, however, it is recognized that articular cartilage is a dynamic system capable of remodeling under functional demands, and of turning over extracellular matrix components. This suggests the existence of a presumably enzymatically mediated "internal remodeling system", controlled by chondrocytes. The chondrocytes produce precisely regulated amounts of proteases and protease inhibitors to induce normal turnover of extracellular matrix components. Under normal conditions, the chondrocytes maintain a balanced extracellular matrix by equating anabolic and catabolic processes, i.e., synthesis and degradation.[11] However, when this balance is disturbed, either by local or systemic factors, cartilage degradation ensues.[22]

Proteases, cytokines, growth factors, and arachidonic acid metabolites all play a role in the pathogenesis of osteoarthrosis. A unique initiating factor, if one exists, has not yet been identified. The finding of one or more of these factors in the synovial fluid or cartilage is not pathognomonic for osteoarthrosis, because all of these factors can also be found in several other pathologic conditions, including inflammation, trauma, and allergy. Therefore, the mere presence of one or more of these factors in the osteoarthrotic temporomandibular joint has little clinical value.

Classification of temporomandibular joint signs and symptoms has until now been based on the stages of internal derangement.[29] However, in many cases these signs and symptoms are attributable to osteoarthrosis.[24] Especially in studies of proteases, cytokines, growth factors, and arachidonic acid metabolites, as well as in studies of cartilage degradation products present in the synovial fluid, findings should be related to the degree of degradation of articular cartilage and to the degree of synovitis, rather than to the stage of internal derangement. Consequently, a classification of temporomandibular joint osteoarthrosis should be based on the degree of cartilage degradation and of synovitis. Degradation of articular cartilage could be divided into four stages: an initial and repair stage, an early stage, an intermediate stage, and a late stage of osteoarthrosis. In our opinion, temporomandibular joint osteoarthrosis is a multifactorial disorder, with various pathogenic pathways, in which several stages of internal derangement may be found. Each stage of internal derangement should be diagnosed as a separate entity.

Conclusions

Primary osteoarthrosis may result in degenerative changes, disc displacement and eventually in changes in joint morphology. All signs and symptoms seem to be the result of this primary, idiopathic process. In secondary osteoarthrosis, degenerative changes are present due to joint afflictions such as rheumatoid arthritis, but may also occur due to disc displacement, or joint hypermobility. The pathology of temporomandibular joint osteoarthrosis involves synovial joint pathology and, basically, connective tissue diseases.

Cartilage matrix degradation is the subject of extensive biochemical research. Several proteases, protease inhibitors, cytokines, and growth factors seem to be involved in the cartilage matrix degradation processes, and affect cartilage, bone, and synovium.

It is becoming increasingly obvious that enzymatic pathways, in addition to mechanical factors, are involved in cartilage matrix degradation. To establish an effective regimen of therapy to decrease the extent of joint destruction, it is important to understand how matrix degradation develops and what enzymes mediate the process. Future research should primarily focus on the biochemics of temporomandibular joint osteoarthrosis.

References

1 de Bont LGM, Stegenga B. Pathology of temporomandibular joint internal derangement and osteoarthrosis. Int J Oral Maxillofac Surg 1993; 22:71

2 Mankin HJ. Clinical features of osteoarthritis. In: Kelley WN, Harris ED, Ruddy S, Sledge CB (eds). Textbook of Rheumatology. 3rd ed. Philadelphia: Saunders, 1989; 1480

3 Hough AJ, Sokoloff L. Pathology of osteoarthritis. In: McCarty DJ (ed). Arthritis and Allied Conditions. A Textbook of Rheumatology. 11th ed, Philadelphia: Lea & Febiger, 1989; 1571

4 Mankin HJ, Brandt KD. Biochemistry and metabolism of articular cartilage in osteoarthritis. In: Moskowitz RW, Howell DS, Goldberg VM, Mankin HJ (eds). Osteoarthritis: Diagnosis and Medical/Surgical Management. 2nd ed. Philadelphia: Saunders 1992; 109

5 de Bont LGM, Boering G, Liem RSB, Eulderink F, Westesson P-L et al. Osteoarthritis and internal derangement of the temporomandibular joint. A light microscopic study. J Oral Maxillofac Surg 1986; 44:634

6 de Bont LGM, Liem RSB, Boering G. Ultrastructure of the articular cartilage of the mandibular condyle: ageing and degeneration. Oral Surg Oral Med Oral Pathol 1985; 60:631

7 de Bont LGM, Boering G, Liem RSB, Havinga P. Osteoarthritis of the temporomandibular joint: a light microscopic and scanning electron microscopic study of the articular cartilage of the mandibular condyle. J Oral Maxillofac Surg 1985; 43:481

8 de Bont LGM, Stegenga B. Terminology for normal findings. In: Clark GT, Sanders B, Bertolami C (eds). Advances in diagnostic and surgical arthroscopy of the temporomandibular joint. Philadelphia: Saunders 1993; 3

9 de Bont LGM, Boering G, Havinga P, Liem RSB. Spatial arrangement of collagen fibrils in the articular cartilage of the mandibular condyle: a LM and SEM study. J Oral Maxillofac Surg 1984; 42:306

10 de Bont LGM, Stegenga B, Boering G. Normal physiology of synovial joints. Articular cartilage. In: Thomas M, Bronstein SL (eds). Arthroscopy of the Temporomandibular Joint. Philadelphia: Saunders 1991; 28

11 Dijkgraaf LC, de Bont LGM, Boering G, Liem RSB. Normal cartilage: structure, biochemistry and metabolism: A review of the literature. J Oral Maxillofac Surg 1995; 53:924.

12 Werb Z. Proteinases and matrix degradation. In: Kelley WN, Harris ED, Ruddy S, Sledge CB (eds). Textbook of Rheumatology. 3rd ed. Philadelphia: Saunders 1989; 300

13 Dean DD, Martel-Pelletier J, Pelletier JP, Howell DS, Woessner JF Jr. et al. Evidence for metalloproteinase and metalloproteinase inhibitor (TIMP) imbalance in human osteoarthritic cartilage. J Clin Invest 1989; 84:678

14 Howell DS, Treadwell BV, Trippel SB. Etiopathogenesis of osteoarthritis. In: Moskowitz RW,

Howell DS, Goldberg VM, Mankin JH (eds). Osteoarthritis: diagnosis and medical/surgical management. 2nd ed. Phialadelphia: Saunders, 1992; 233

15 Pelletier JP, Roughley PJ, DiBattista JA, McCollum R, Martel-Pelletier J et al. Are cytokines involved in osteoarthritic pathophysiology? Semin Arthritis Rheum 1991; 20:12

16 Goetzl EJ, Goldstein IM. Arachidonic acid metabolites. In: McCarty DJ (ed). Arthritis and allied conditions. A textbook of rheumatology. 11th ed. Philadelphia, Lea & Febiger, 1989; 409

17 Lewis RA. Prostaglandins and leukotrienes. In: Kelley WN, Harris ED, Ruddy S, Sledge CB (eds). Textbook of Rheumatology. 3rd ed. Philadelphia: Saunders, 1989; 253

18 Howell DS. Etiopathogenesis of osteoarthritis. In: McCarty DJ (ed). Arthritis and allied conditions. A textbook of rheumatology. 11th ed. Philadelphia: Lea & Febiger, 1989; 1595

19 Freeman MAR, Meachim G. Ageing and degeneration. In: Freeman MAR (ed). Adult articular cartilage. 2nd ed. London: Pitman, 1979; 487–540

20 Dijkgraaf LC, de Bont LGM, Boering G, Liem RSB. Normal synovial membrane of the temporomandibular joint. A review of the literature. Part II. Function, biochemistry and metabolism. J Oral Maxillofac Surg 1996; In press.

21 Dijkgraaf LC, de Bont LGM, Boering G, Liem RSB. Normal synovial membrane of the temporomandibular joint. A review of the literature. Part I. Structure. J Oral Maxillofac Surg 1996; In press.

22 Dijkgraaf LC, de Bont LGM, Boering G, Liem RSB. The structure, biochemistry, and metabolism of osteoarthritic cartilage: A review of the literature. J Oral Maxillofac Surg 1995; 53:1182.

23 Stegenga B, de Bont LGM, Boering G, van Willigen JD. Tissue responses to degenerative changes in the temporomandibular joint: a review. J Oral Maxillofac Surg 1991; 49:1079

24 Stegenga B, de Bont LGM, Boering G. Osteoarthrosis as the cause of craniomandibular pain and dysfunction: a unifying concept. J Oral Maxillofac Surg 1989; 47:249

25 de Bont LGM, Stegenga B, Boering G. Hard tissue pathology. Osteoarthrosis. In: Thomas M, Bronstein SL (eds). Arthroscopy of the temporomandibular joint. Philadelphia: Saunders 1991; 258

26 Schellhas KP, Wilkes CH, Fritts HM, et al. MR of osteochondritis dissecans and avascular necrosis of the mandibular condyle. AJR 1989; 152:551

27 Stegenga B, de Bont LGM, Boering G. A proposed classification of temporomandibular disorders based on synovial joint pathology. J Craniomandibular Pract 1989; 7:107

28 Kircos LT, Ortendahl DA, Mark AS, Arakawa M. Magnetic resonance imaging of the TMJ disc in asymptomatic volunteers. J Oral Maxillofac Surg 1987; 45:852

29 Wilkes CH. Internal derangement of the temporomandibular joint: pathologic variations. Arch Otolaryngol Head Neck Surg 1989; 115:469

Management of Temporomandibular
Joint Degenerative Diseases
ed. by B. Stegenga & L.G.M. de Bont
© 1996 Birkhäuser Verlag Basel/Switzerland

Temporomandibular joint degenerative diseases: clinical diagnosis

Boudewijn Stegenga

Department of Oral and Maxillofacial Surgery, University Hospital Groningen, 9700 RB Groningen, The Netherlands

Summary: Pathologic changes of the temporomandibular joint basically represent synovial joint pathology, and it is therefore logical to base the descriptors for disorders of this joint on the nomenclature used for joints elsewhere in the body. In this chapter, basic diagnostic terms and terms used to describe pathologic mechanisms are defined. A systematic approach to arrive at a diagnosis providing a comprehensive basis for treatment is discussed.

Introduction

Diagnostic assessment is an important step in the management and evaluation of treatment outcome of temporomandibular disorders of all types. Especially in painful disorders where surgery is under consideration, it is important to identify the pathologic processes and their clinical manifestations, as well as factors that may influence the decision-making process of diagnosis and treatment planning. A uniform diagnostic approach requires agreement about

- the terminology used to designate temporomandibular disorders
- underlying pathologic mechanisms and clinical manifestations
- a comprehensive diagnostic strategy.

All of these issues involve controversial elements that are addressed in this chapter.

Terminology

The widely accepted term to designate disorders of the mandibular locomotor system, involving the craniomandibular articulation and its actuating musculature, is 'temporomandibular disorders'.[1-3] The craniomandibular articulation consists of two temporomandibular joints, each showing all the basic characteristics of a synovial joint with an articular disc. Pathologic changes of the temporomandibular joint are basically synovial joint pathology, and it is therefore logical to base the descriptors for disorders of this joint on the nomenclature used for joints elsewhere in the body.[2]

Classification

Disorders of the mandibular locomotor apparatus may originate within the joint (arthropathies) or be non-articular. The disorder may be the result of loco-regional pathology or be part of a more generalized disorder. The major groups of synovial joint disorders are inflammatory and non-inflammatory arthropathies. The non-articular temporomandibular disorders most commonly involve neuromuscular disorders, although other disorders may also be the cause of temporomandibular pain or movement disturbances. The distinction between arthropathies and non-articular disorders is different from the commonly made distinction between 'arthrogenic' and 'myogenic' pain or dysfunction. These terms reflect manifestations of temporomandibular disorders rather than the disorder itself.

Inflammatory arthropathies
The common term for an inflammatory joint disorder is arthritis. Temporomandibular joint arthritis may be due to systemic conditions, e.g., rheumatoid arthritis, or more localized conditions related to trauma, infection, or degenerative changes (table 1).

Table 1. Classification of arthropathies

Inflammatory arthropathies (arthritis)	Non-inflammatory arthropathies
Primary arthritis	
rheumatoid arthritis	Osteoarthrosis
juvenile arthritis	primary
HLA-B27 associated arthritis	secondary
ankylosing spondylitis	Internal joint derangement
psoriatic arthritis	Aseptic necrosis
Reiter's syndrome	Synovial chondromatosis
Secondary arthritis	
Infective and infection-associated arthritis	
traumatic arthritis	
crystal-induced arthritis	
degenerative arthritis (osteoarthritis)	

Synovitis refers to inflammation of the synovial membrane. It results in an escape of fluid into the joint cavity (effusion), and alterations in the composition of the synovial fluid. When severe, necrosis and fibrin deposition on the synovial surfaces may cause adhesions, which reduce the joint space and eventually may lead to fibrous ankylosis.

Capsulitis describes inflammation of the outer layer of the capsule. It is characterized by pain with capsular stretching. Clinically, capsulitis is indistinguishable from synovitis.[4] Most commonly, capsulitis results from stretching the capsule beyond its physiological range, e.g., due to habits or local trauma. During the healing process, the capsule may adhere to adjacent tissue (adhesive capsulitis) or heal in a shortened state (capsular fibrosis).

Non-inflammatory arthropathies

Non-inflammatory disorders refer to disorders in which joint dysfunction occurs in the absence of overt inflammation (table 1). Osteoarthrosis is the most common degenerative disease of synovial joints. It primarily affects the articular cartilage, probably due to its limited adaptive capacity compared with other connective tissues, and the subchondral bone. Primary osteoarthrosis develops in the absence of any known underlying predisposing factor; in secondary osteoarthrosis, an underlying local or systemic pathogenetic factor, e.g., trauma, prior surgery, recurrent dislocation, crystal deposition disorders, avascular necrosis, or post-inflammation cartilage damage, can be identified.

Chondromalacia is a term originally used to describe local softening of the cartilage of the patella and is now increasingly applied to describe the degenerative changes occurring in articular cartilage of the temporomandibular joint.[5] Internal derangement is an orthopedic term, defined as a localized mechanical fault in a synovial joint which interferes with its smooth action.[6] In the temporomandibular joint, internal derangements are commonly observed in combination with osteoarthrosis.[7] Chondromalacia starts focally in the joint. When progressive, it may affect the frictional characteristics of the articular surfaces to an extent that it produces clinical manifestations. Since the various tissues of the temporomandibular joint lie in immediate juxtaposition to one another, compensatory and protective responses in the adjacent tissues and associated musculature occur rather early in the disease.[8] In other words, early degenerative changes may progress to compensatory and pathologic tissue responses that frequently become clinically manifest as internal derangements.

Osteoarthritis includes an inflammatory component, presumably caused by waste products from the degenerative changes and inflammatory mediators released in the joint cavity. By definition, osteoarthritis (osteoarthrosis in conjuction with synovitis) is a secondary inflammatory arthropathy.

Clinical manifestations

Like all disorders of the locomotor apparatus, temporomandibular disorders are characterized by pain and movement disturbances. Thus, pain assessment and identifying disturbances in mandibular movement form the basic elements of the clinical examination. The pain is of the musculoskeletal type, originates in the joint (arthralgia) or in the muscles that power the joints (myalgia), and relates directly to masticatory function.[9,10] Movement disturbances may present as restrictions of or interferences during mandibular movements.

The findings during the clinical examination are summarized in a 'working diagnosis', providing information about the extent of the disorder, etiologic and contributing factors, pain, mandibular movement characteristics, and evidence for internal joint derangements.

Extent of the disorder

It is essential to know whether the disorder is confined to the mandibular locomotor apparatus or whether there is evidence that the temporomandibular arthropathy is part of a more generalized disease.[2]

Contributing factors

The initiation and continuation of the disorder may be related to biologic factors (e.g., the patient's general health, traumatic injuries, previous surgery, orthognathic treatment), behavioural factors (e.g., chewing habits, bruxism, posture), and psychosocial factors.[11]

Pain diagnosis

Pain history and clinical examination
An important aspect of history taking is to obtain an accurate description of the pain complaint, comprising information about the anatomic locations of the pain, its onset and manner of flow, whether or not the pain is induced by certain activities, its intensity, and its impact on the patient. The course of the pain complaint and how it relates to other signs and symptoms should be described. A pain questionnaire is helpful in obtaining a comprehensive description of the pain history.[9]

The clinical examination aims at determining whether the pain emanates primarily from the joint or from the masticatory muscles. The joints are tested for tenderness during active mandibular movements, palpation, and manipulation (i.e., compression, distraction, and passive movements).[12] The regional muscles are tested by palpation and by selective contraction.[12] Most directly, the source of pain and whether it is primary or referred can be identified by applying local anesthesia.[13,14]

Pain characteristics
Pain related to temporomandibular disorders is acute, subacute, or persistent musculoskeletal pain. The pain typically relates intimately to biomechanical function and responds proportionately to provocation.[10] In case of persistent pain, one should always be aware of a chronic pain syndrome requiring special management.

Arthralgia primarily originates from the joint ligaments (i.e., capsule and disc attachments), and subchondral bone. Ligamentous nociceptors are high-threshold mechanoreceptors. They are stimulated when the ligament is stretched beyond its functional range. However, inflammatory mediators may lower the pain threshold, making nociceptors more sensitive to stimulation. As a result, stimulation from normal functioning may initiate sensations of discomfort. Thus, discomfort resulting from manual palpation or functional manipulation of the joint is indicative of an inflammatory joint condition. Intermittent pain associated with other symptoms of interference should be interpreted as being due to significant noxious strain being placed momentarily on the ligament. Similarly, bone pain may be elicited by mechanical stimulation of nociceptors, for example, during frictional movement.[5]

Arthralgia usually exerts a protective inhibitory influence on biomechanical activity. This is a physiologic mechanism of skeletal muscles, initiated by altered proprioceptive, sensory, or nociceptive input to the central nervous system. The term 'muscle splinting' is frequently used because the muscles that flex and extend the joint simultaneously contract.[15] Muscle splinting in itself may become symptomatic, presenting as local muscle tenderness especially on contraction, and muscle weakness. Sometimes this phenomenon is erroneously termed 'muscle spasm', which is a centrally induced muscle contraction (cramp) giving rise to acute pain, increased electromyographic activity, and muscle rigidity or shortening.[16] Another common type of muscle pain is myofascial pain, which may occur loco-regionally or as part of a generalized condition (fibromyalgia).[16] The muscle contains a localized hyperirritable spot (myofascial trigger point) that is painful on compression and can evoke a referred pain pattern. In addition, stiffness after inactivity, resistance to stretch, palpable hardenings within the muscle, and muscle weakness may be presenting symptoms.[16,17]

Mandibular movement characteristics

Joint as well as muscle dysfunction may cause alterations of mandibular movement patterns. The ranges of active mandibular movements in all directions (opening, protrusive and lateral excursions) are useful clinical measures. As a rule of thumb, an approximate 4:1 ratio between the range of maximal opening and lateral excursion to the side opposite the affected joint has been suggested by Farrar and McCarty as an indication of 'normal',[18] although one should be aware of a considerable variability. Additional information is provided by measuring the range of opening after passive stretch. Regarding the path of opening, any deflection or deviation from a straight midline movement should be noted and recorded.

Movement restriction of muscular origin usually affects mouth opening without appreciably affecting protrusion or lateral excursion.[19] Thus, muscle restriction alone tends to decrease the ratio between maximal opening and lateral excursion. Associated myalgia may occur with passive stretching beyond maximal active mouth opening, and with contraction.

When the joint capsule becomes less extensible, e.g., due to capsulitis or capsular fibrosis, it imposes a premature limitation of the translatory movement of the disc-condyle assembly. Also, several intra-capsular conditions may arrest translatory movement within the joint. This causes restriction of mandibular movement on opening and on contralateral excursion, usually combined with a mandibular midline deflection with opening and with protrusion. The most common causes include permanent anterior disc displacement and adhesion formation.

Internal joint derangements

An internal derangement is an intra-articular mechanical disturbance which interferes with the joint's smooth action.[6] Symptoms and signs include subjective sensations of sticking or catching, joint noises (clicking and crepitus being the most common), and interferences during normal translatory movement usually in conjunction with deviations of the incisal path. A discrete clicking sound represents the moment that an obstruction is overcome, e.g., the release of a temporary fixation of articular surfaces, overriding of a structural irregularity of the articular surface or a loose body, or reduction of an anteriorly displaced disc. When the obstruction cannot be overcome, 'locking' is experienced, which usually causes a restricted range of movement.

Frictional disc hesitation and adhesions

Jaw inactivity causes protracted arrested movement between opposing articular surfaces. In the absence of movement, the synovial fluid tends to become more viscid ('gelation phenomenon'),[20] and lubrication is exhausted. Increased friction tends to immobilize the disc against the articular eminence (frictional disc hesitation).[21] Attempts at resuming activity may cause a sticking sensation. When the obstruction is overcome, a non-reproducible clicking sound is released, and pain due to momentary stretching of the disc attachment may occur. This may be more pronounced when clenching has accompanied the inactive period. Prolonged immobility allows intra-articular adhesions to form and mature, eventually leading to obliteration of the joint cavity.

Structural surface irregularities

Structural irregularities of the articulating surfaces, resulting from growth disturbances, trauma, remodeling, or osteoarthrotic changes, may also interfere with smooth functioning. Characteristically, the symptoms are discrete and reproducible as similar movements are executed.[22] Reciprocal symptoms during opening and closing occur at the same point of the translatory movement. Frequently, deviations of the midline occur as a compensatory mechanism.[23] More pronounced structural irregularities are part of arthrotic changes, which may eventually produce crepitus.

Disc displacement

Disc displacements are the most commonly known internal derangements. Basically, disc displacement is permitted by stretching of the attachments that bind the disc to the condyle, and by thinning of the posterior band of the disc.

These events are more frequently caused by frictional movement due to early degenerative changes of the articular cartilage (i.e., chondromalacia) than is usually assumed. Stretching of disc attachments accounts for a relative hypermobility in the lower joint compartment. In a 'classical' reducing disc displacement, the disc reduces relative to both the condyle and the articular eminence, producing a clicking sound. With time, the retrodiscal tissue tends to become less elastic and more fibrous, which causes the reduction to occur later in the traject of translation. Moreover, the condyle repetitively pushes against the posterior band of the disc, which causes the disc to gradually deform in response to the loading pattern. In other words, with time reduction is achieved with more and more difficulty. In addition, a relative hypomobility of the disc developes in the upper joint compartment. In some patients adhesions may develop under these circumstances. This causes reduction to occur only relative to the condyle, which may clinically present as a translatory restriction of a clicking joint. The translation that occurs takes place in the lower compartment.[24]

A 'closed-lock' clinical picture is characterized by absence of clicking and by restriction of translatory movement. When the patient is able to unlock the jaw either actively or by auto-manipulation, clicking recommences and the mouth can be opened without restriction. This transitional condition can be termed 'semi-permanent disc displacement'.[25] A recent onset of locking which can only be unlocked by manipulation by the examiner is indicative of an acute permanent disc displacement (acute closed-lock). Typically, in this locking stage the joint may suddenly be mobilized, which makes the formation of intra-articular adhesions unlikely.

A permanent disc displacement develops with time from a state of obvious obstruction of condylar translation by the displaced disc to only slight restriction of the translatory capacity of the joint. This natural course may be explained by gradual stretching of the disc attachments without developing adhesions.[26] Persistent restriction of movement is usually the result of adhesion formation. When the disc is permanently out of place, the retrodiscal tissue is permanently loaded. In this situation, the joint tends to adapt by remodeling, compensating for the displaced disc, which, at the same time, progressively deforms. Continued overloading may, however, overrule this compensating mechanism, giving rise to decompensation characterized by perforation or even laceration of the retrodiscal tissue. In general, the later stages of the disorder are clinically characterized by mild residual symptoms, such as some crepitus and possibly a mild restricted opening. In a decompensated joint coarse crepitus is frequently heard, and pain episodes are easily caused by continuation of contributing factors that overload the joint. We termed this late stage 'residual osteoarthrosis' to indicate that osteoarthrotic changes had already started in previous stages of internal derangement, possibly from the very beginning of the process.[25]

Subluxation and luxation
Another type of internal derangement may occur when the disc-condyle assembly 'jumps' across the articular eminence (subluxation).[27] The condition where

the condyle gets stuck in front of the articular eminence resulting in an inability to close the mouth after opening wide is referred to as luxation.[2]

Staging temporomandibular joint internal derangements
Apart from specifying the internal derangement by indicating what mechanical interferences or restrictions exist, it may be useful to put the internal derangement into a time frame. The most recent, and widely applied, staging system has been drawn up by Wilkes (table 2).[28] This staging system has been extended for imaging and arthroscopic characteristics.[29,30]

Table 2. Wilkes' staging of temporomandibular joint internal derangements

Stage		Characteristics
I	early	no pain or restriction of motion reciprocal clicking on/after loading (eating) slight anterior disc displacement on imaging
II	early/intermediate	reciprocal clicking, periodic locking mild to moderate pain episodes, joint tenderness altered disc position on imaging
III	intermediate	multiple episodes of pain, joint tenderness intermittent and sustained locking, restricted movement altered disc position, disc deformation on imaging variable adhesions
IV	intermediate/late	chronic pain, variable severe episodes variable restriction of movement altered position and shape of disc hard tissue changes condylar shape altered on imaging multiple adhesions
V	late	variable episodic pain chronic restricted movement gross crepitus anterior disc displacement, altered morphology, perforation gross anatomic deformity

The early stage shows the characteristics of an early reducing disc displacement. In the early/intermediate stage the first few episodes of pain occur, along with increased intensity of clicking sounds, fitting the clinical characteristics of an advanced reducing disc displacement. In the intermediate stage, major mechanical symptoms such as transient and sustained locking, marked restriction of motion, and multiple episodes of pain and tenderness occur. This stage is equivalent with a diagnosis of subacute permanent disc displacement. The intermediate/late stage shows the characteristics of a chronic permanent disc displacement, with variable pain and restriction of motion, depending on the extent of disc displacement and deformity, and on the presence of adhesions. According to Wilkes' staging, perforation of the retrodiscal tissue (clinically characterized by crepitus and variable pain) is the characteristic feature of late stage internal derangement.

Wilkes' staging system covers the most common sequence of events reflecting the natural history of osteoarthrosis and internal derangement of the temporomandibular joint.[26] However, numerous variations in this time frame occur. These variations not only relate to the position of the disc but also include other forms of internal derangement, mentioned earlier. It appears to be realistic to take pathologic mechanisms other than disc displacement into account as well. With increasing understanding of pathologic mechanisms, osteoarthrosis is currently considered to result from an altered cartilage metabolism, not necessarily related to mechanical factors, causing release of proteolytic enzymes capable of degrading the cartilage matrix. When attempts at repair fail to keep pace with the degradative activity, cartilage breakdown continues. Symptoms, i.e., pain and mechanical derangements, occur later in the course of the disease. Based on these pathologic processes, the course of osteoarthrosis can be staged. Emphasizing differences in the clinical picture may easily lead to over-specification. On the other hand, denying differences could have therapeutic consequences. We attempted to find a balance between the number of specific diagnostic entities and treatment approaches, which resulted in our modification of the traditional stages of osteoarthrosis (table 3).[25] Future research should further relate clinical subgroups to pathologic changes and indicators thereof.

Table 3. Diagnostic stages of osteoarthrosis and internal derangement

I	chondromalacia non-adhesive — adhesive

II	reducing disc displacement
	    early — advanced
	    non-adhesive — adhesive

III	locking
	    semi-reducing disc displacement (clicking, intermittent locking)
	    semi-permanent disc displacement (closed lock, unlocking actively possible)
	    acute closed-lock (unlocking only by passive manipulation)

IV	non-reducing (permanent) disc displacement
	    (sub)acute — chronic
	    non-adhesive — adhesive
	    compensated — decompensated

V	residual osteoarthrosis compensated — decompensated

Proposed strategy for diagnosing temporomandibular disorders

Classification: differential diagnosis

Classification of the disorder is based on the descriptive information provided by the working diagnosis. Important issues include:

−   Are the symptoms and signs confined to the mandibular locomotor system or is there evidence for a more systemic basis as part of a diffuse connective tissue disorder?
−   Do the symptoms and signs primarily reflect an arthropathy or a non-articular disorder? Do the symptoms and signs primarily reflect a degenerative, growth-related, or inflammatory disorder? In degenerative disorders, internal derangements dominate the clinical picture, i.e., most of the complaints relate to mechanical interferences during or restriction of movements. Growth-related disorders (developmental, acquired, neoplastic) frequently are non-symptomatic, or become symptomatic when the disorder interferes with normal functioning. In arthritis, pain is the dominating symptom. It is characteristically continuous, aggravated by functioning, and has secondary muscle effects.
−   Do secondary processes modify the clinical picture? Examples include capsular fibrosis, ankylosis, inflammation secondary to a non-inflammatory disorder (e.g., osteoarthritis), degeneration secondary to inflammatory disorders (e.g., osteoarthrosis secondary to rheumatoid arthritis or crystal deposition diseases), or secondary muscular phenomena (myofascial pain, muscle splinting, muscle contracture, tendomyositis).

Specification: disease-specific diagnosis

Within each category, specific diagnostic entities can be distinguished. To identify the disorder(s) that account for the patient's symptoms and signs, the presence or absence of characteristic features of the disorders contained in the differential diagnosis must be verified. Frequently, additional diagnostic information (e.g., additional radiographs, computerized tomography, magnetic resonance imaging, bone scanning, laboratory tests, diagnostic arthroscopy, psychological evaluation, external consultations) is necessary.

Only a few disorders have been defined by specific diagnostic criteria.[25,31] Much work remains to be done in this field in order to obtain sufficient uniformity. Based on their natural course, some disorders may be further characterized by putting them in a time frame (staging).

Individualization: patient-specific diagnosis

Patients with the same specific diagnosis based on the presence of defining criteria likely differ in other respects. These factors may account for differences in response to therapeutic intervention. For several disorders, the age of disease onset or presentation may be an important distinguishing factor. Patients may differ with regard to the factors contributing to their symptoms. Differences usually involve pain perception and behaviour, function impairment, and general well-being. In fact, these variables reflect the impact of the disorder on the individual and the patient's ability to cope with it. Such information is required for predicting and also for evaluating the treatment outcome. Thus, patient-specific information is added to the disease-specific diagnosis, in terms of the disorder's impact on the individual (including pain impact specification, function impairment).

Discussion

According to the presented strategy, a disease-specific diagnosis is based on measurable criteria (such as range of motion, joint noises, deviations, radiographic changes) and presenting subjective signs (such as pain). It is combined with the disorder's impact on the individual as expressed in the patient's subjective complaints. This is an essential aspect in relation to treatment planning and prognosis, since the individual status determines the extent of suffering from the underlying disease.

During the course of temporomandibular joint degenerative diseases, degradative enzymes affect the integrity of the articular cartilage, elicit responses of the synovial membrane altering the synovial fluid, and produce changes in subchondral bone, the disc, and the joint capsule.[8] Each joint component may be affected and should, therefore, be examined to establish a comprehensive diagnosis and a solid basis for treatment planning. Directing treatment to only one aspect of the disease process may be a common reason for treatment failure related to an incomplete diagnosis. Moreover, failure to recognize or address extra-articular manifestations of the disorder or concomitant disorders (myofascial pain, chronic pain syndrome) are common reasons for treatment failure.

Several common treatment procedures are aimed at restoring disc position. However, with the knowledge available today, it seems that these procedures are only justified in cases in which the degenerative process is still in an early stage without major changes in the shape of the disc, enabling repair following restoration of joint anatomy. The reparability of the articular disc must at least be questioned in a joint that has a long history of clicking, and characteristic features of advanced reducing or permanent disc displacement. Magnetic resonance imaging has contributed considerably to our appreciation of the significance of disc displacement in relation to other clinical symptoms and pathologic mechanisms. There appears to be a considerable interindividual variability with regard to the position of the disc. Asymptomatic joints may appear to have a displaced disc, and, conversely, patients with a clinical diagnosis of internal derangement may appear to have a 'normally' positioned disc.[32] The presence of joint sounds that have not changed over an extended period of time indicates that the structures involved have adapted and these joints should, therefore, be considered 'normal'.[8] The presence of joint sounds does not necessarily indicate treatment failure. Also, it must be appreciated that detection of a displaced disc by imaging does not necessarily indicate joint pathology justifying treatment.

Summary and conclusion

A specific clinical diagnosis of temporomandibular disorders should be based on a comprehensive examination summarized in a working diagnosis. The major elements of the working diagnosis include the disorder's clinical symptoms and signs reflecting the possible underlying pathologic changes.

A differential diagnosis is made by identifying the main category or categories of temporomandibular disorders that is/are compatible with the working diagnosis. At this point, it is important to assess the extent of the disorder (loco-regional, generalized, systemic), its primary source (articular, non-articular) and nature (degenerative, inflammatory, growth related), and to identify secondary pathologic processes going on. To specifically identify the disorder(s) that account for the patient's clinical manifestations, the presence or absence of characteristic features of the disorders contained in the differential diagnosis must be verified, if necessary by carrying out additional diagnostic examinations.

Although clinical and imaging characteristics determine the diagnosis, the extent of pain and function impairment as well as other more patient-specific factors determine the need for, modality, prognosis, and outcome of treatment. Therefore, the final essential step in diagnosing temporomandibular disorders is to add this patient-specific information to the disease-specific diagnosis.

References

1 Bell WE. Classification of temporomandibular disorders. In: Laskin DM, Greenfield W, Gale E, et al. (eds). The president's conference on the examination, diagnosis and management of temporomandibular disorders. Chicago: American Dental Association, 1983
2 Stegenga B. Classification of temporomandibular disorders based on synovial joint pathology. In: Stegenga B. Temporomandibular joint osteoarthrosis and internal derangement: diagnostic and therapeutic outcome assessment. Thesis, University of Groningen, The Netherlands, 1991; 40
3 McNeill CH (ed). Current controversies in temporomandibular disorders. Chicago: Quintessence, 1992; 17
4 Bell WE. Temporomandibular disorders. Classification, diagnosis and management. 3rd ed. Chicago: Yearbook Med Publ, 1990; 339
5 Quinn JHL. Pathogenesis of temporomandibular joint chondromalacia and arthralgia. Oral Maxillofac Surg Clin North Am 1989; 1:47

6 Adams JC, Hamblen DL. Outline of orthopedics. 11th ed. Edinburgh: Churchill Livingstone, 1990
7 de Bont LGM, Boering G, Liem RSB, Eulderink F, Westesson P-L et al. Osteoarthrosis and internal derangement of the temporomandibular joint. A light microscopic study. J Oral Maxillofac Surg 1986; 44:634
8 Stegenga B, de Bont LGM, Boering G, van Willigen JD. Tissue responses to degenerative changes of the temporomandibular joint. A review. J Oral Maxillofac Surg 1991; 49:1079
9 Stegenga B, de Bont LGM, Boering G. Temporomandibular joint pain assessment. J Orofacial Pain 1993; 7:23
10 Bell WE. Orofacial pains. 4th ed. Chicago: Yearbook Med Publ, 1989; 108
11 Fricton JR, Chung SC. Contributing factors. In: Fricton JR, Kroening RJ, Hathaway KM (eds). TMJ and craniofacial pain: diagnosis and management. St. Louis: Ishiyaku EuroAmerica, 1988
12 Friedman MH, Weisberg J. Temporomandibular disorders. Diagnosis and treatment. Chicago: Quintessence, 1985; 43
13 Kaplan AS. Examination and diagnosis. In: Kaplan AS, Assael LA (eds) Temporomandibular disorders: diagnosis and treatment. Philadelphia: Saunders, 1991; 304
14 Mahan PE, Alling CC. Facial pain. 3rd ed. Philadelphia: Lea & Febiger, 1991; 82
15 Mahan PE, Alling CC. Facial pain. 3rd ed. Philadelphia: Lea & Febiger, 1991; 134
16 Fricton JR, Kroening RJ, Haley D. Muscular disorders. In: Fricton JR, Kroening RJ, Hathaway KM (eds). TMJ and craniofacial pain: diagnosis and management. St. Louis: Ishiyaku EuroAmerica, 1988
17 Travell JG, Simons DG. Myofascial pain and dysfunction. The trigger point manual. Baltimore: Williams & Wilkins, 1983
18 Farrar WB, McCarty WL. A clinical outline of temporomandibular joint diagnosis and treatment. 7th ed. Montgomery: Normandie, 1982
19 Bell WE. Temporomandibular disorders. Classification, diagnosis and management. 3rd ed. Chicago: Yearbook Med Publ, 1990; 145
20 Frost HM. Musculoskeletal pain. In: Alling CC, Mahan PE (eds). Facial pain. 2nd ed. Philadelphia: Lea & Febiger, 1977
21 Ogus H. The mandibular joint: internal rearrangement. Br J Oral Maxillofac Surg 1987; 25:218
22 Mahan PE, Alling CC. Facial pain. 3rd ed. Philadelphia: Lea & Febiger, 1991; 210
23 Bell WE. Temporomandibular disorders. Classification, diagnosis and management. 3rd ed. Chicago: Yearbook Med Publ, 1990; 155
24 Moses JJ. Lateral impingement syndrome and endaural surgical technique. Oral Maxillofac Surg Clin North Am 1989; 1:165
25 Stegenga B, de Bont LGM, Boering G. Classification of osteoarthrosis and internal derangement of the temporomandibular joint. Part II. Specific diagnostic criteria. J Craniomandibular Pract 1992; 10:107
26 Nickerson JW, Boering G. Natural course of osteoarthrosis as it relates to internal derangement of the temporomandibular joint. Oral Maxillofac Surg Clin North Am 1989; 1:27
27 Mahan PE, Alling CC. Facial pain. 3rd ed. Philadelphia: Lea & Febiger, 1991; 207
28 Wilkes CH. Internal derangement of the temporomandibular joint: pathologic variations. Arch Otolaryngol Head Neck Surg 1989; 115:469
29 Schellhas KP. Internal derangement of the temporomandibular joint: radiologic staging with clinical, surgical, and pathologic correlation. Magn Resonance Imag 1989; 7:495
30 Bronstein SL. Guidelines for temporomandibular joint arthroscopy. In: Thomas M, Bronstein SL. Arthroscopy of the temporomandibular joint. Philadelphia: Saunders, 1991; 229
31 Stegenga B. Temporomandibular joint osteoarthrosis and internal derangement. Diagnostic and therapeutic outcome assessment. Thesis, University of Groningen, The Netherlands, 1991; 213–239
32 Kircos L, Ortendahl D, Mark A, Arakawa M. MRI of the TMJ disc in asymptomatic volunteers. J Oral Maxillofac Surg 1987; 45:852

Management of Temporomandibular
Joint Degenerative Diseases
ed. by B. Stegenga & L.G.M. de Bont
© 1996 Birkhäuser Verlag Basel/Switzerland

Temporomandibular joint disc displacement: a re-evaluation of its significance

M. Franklin Dolwick

*University of Florida College of Dentistry, Oral and Maxillofacial Surgery, Gainesville, Florida
32610, USA*

Summary: During the past two decades, disc position has been the focus of classification, diagnosis,
and treatment of temporomandibular joint internal derangement. It was proposed that joint pain,
mandibular dysfunction, osteoarthrosis, and growth disturbances were caused by disc displacement.
Arthroscopic observation and treatment outcomes of arthroscopy and arthrocentesis have provided new
insights into the pathology of temporomandibular joint internal derangements. Recent evidence indicates
that the role of disc displacement as the primary pathologic factor may not be justified. Internal
derangement is much more complicated than simply disc displacement.

Introduction

The publications by Farrar relating signs and symptoms of mandibular dysfunction to disc displacement, and the rediscovery of arthrography by Wilkes,
stimulated renewed interest in temporomandibular joint internal derangement.[1,2] During the 1970s and 1980s numerous publications documenting disc
displacement and its clinical presentation appeared in the literature.[3-7] Supporting clinical evidence for disc displacement came from diagnostic imaging and
surgical observations correlated with clinical signs and symptoms. It was
proposed that arthralgia, mandibular dysfunction, osteoarthrosis, and mandibular growth disturbances could be attributed to displacement of the temporomandibular joint disc. The position and shape of the disc became the focus of
classification, diagnosis, and treatment of pain and dysfunction. However, in
spite of the clinical evidence supporting the existence of disc displacement,
there remained many unanswered questions which raised doubt as to the
significance of disc displacement.

In 1983, we concluded that displacement of the temporomandibular joint
disc was reality and, further, the major cause of arthralgia, dysfunction, and
osteoarthrosis.[8] During the past decade much has been learned about internal
joint derangements. The purpose of this chapter is to re-evaluate the relationship of disc position to pain, mandibular dysfunction, osteoarthrosis, and
growth disturbances, and thus the significance of disc displacement.

Relationship to pain

Since pain in patients with disc displacement is usually aggravated during movement, it seemed reasonable that the pain originated from pressure and traction on the disc attachments. In joints with anterior disc displacement, the loose, vascular, innervated retrodiscal tissue is displaced between the condyle and fossa and could be compressed or stretched during function. However, there is still the perplexing question why many, perhaps most, patients with disc displacement have no pain while some have severe pain.

Clicking has been shown to occur in 30-50% of the population. Most individuals with clicking joints have some form of disc displacement, yet most of these people do not have pain.[9] The prevalence of clicking is generally found to be evenly distributed between men and women, yet pain is reported much more often by females. It has also been demonstrated that when normal temporomandibular joints, i.e., free of signs and symptoms, are studied arthrographically or with magnetic resonance imaging, approximately 30% of the joints show evidence of disc displacement.[10,11] It has also been observed that when bilateral arthrograms are performed on patients with unilateral symptoms, the non-painful joint demonstrates evidence of disc derangement 88% of the time.[12] The most compelling evidence against the displaced disc as the cause of temporomandibular arthralgia comes from the observations that arthroscopy and arthrocentesis of the superior joint compartment reduces or eliminates pain in patients with closed-lock without repositioning the displaced disc.[13-15] These findings make it obvious that while disc displacement may exist, it is not necessarily related to pain.

Relationship to dysfunction

The relationship of disc displacement to reciprocal clicking, when the clicks occur at different positions during opening and closing movements, is clear, and the evidence supporting this relationship is strong. Using arthrography, it has been demonstrated that during opening the disc is pushed anteriorly until a click occurs, at which time the disc returned to a normal relationship with the condyle.[2,4] It was also observed that during closing, the disc is again displaced anteriorly. Further, the reduction and displacement of the disc correlated with the clinical finding of reciprocal clicking. The anatomic events associated with reciprocal clicking were confirmed by Isberg using high speed cinematography on autopsy specimens.[7]

Temporomandibular joint arthrography performed upon patients with closed-lock demonstrated that the disc was displaced anteriorly and remained displaced throughout the opening and closing cycle of movement.[2,4] This led to the obvious conclusion that the displaced disc was the cause of the observed restricted opening. However, the observations that arthroscopy and arthrocentesis with lavage of the superior joint compartment without repositioning the disc re-established normal mouth opening in patients with closed-lock have seriously questioned this conclusion.[13-15] If normal range of motion can be re-established without repositioning the displaced disc, then alternative explanations for closed-lock are plausible.[16]

Relationship to osteoarthrosis

The relationship of disc displacement to osteoarthrosis is controversial. Studies of human temporomandibular joints have provided evidence that disc displacement is associated with an increased incidence of osteoarthrosis.[6] Osteoarthrosis of the temporomandibular joint has been documented in more than 50% of patients with disc derangement. With imaging studies, osteoarthrosis is rarely observed in joints with normal disc position and is most often observed in joints with disc perforation and severe deformation.[17] These results support the idea that disc displacement precedes osteoarthrosis and that disc displacement may be a cause of osteoarthrosis.

Alternatively, early osteoarthrotic changes such as articular cartilage softening and fibrillation have been observed arthroscopically in the temporomandibular joints with normal disc position or minimally displaced disc. Additionally, de Bont observed histologically "osteoarthrotic changes" affecting the articular surfaces of the temporomandibular joint in four out of eight joints with normal disc-condyle relationships.[18] These results support the idea that osteoarthrotic changes precede disc displacement and that disc displacement may be a sign of osteoarthrosis and not its cause.

While it appears that disc displacement and osteoarthrosis occur together, it is unclear whether disc displacement precedes or follows osteoarthrosis. It is possible that both pathways exist. A displaced disc may cause the development of osteoarthrosis or osteoarthrosis may cause disc displacement. It is also possible that they occur together but are unrelated.

Relationship to growth disturbance

It has recently been stated that disc displacement is a significant cause of growth disturbance.[19] Imaging studies demonstrated disc derangement in association with mandibular deficiency and asymmetry.[20] These studies were reported to support earlier observations by Boering and Ricketts.[21,22] Conversely, not all growing patients who have disc displacement grow abnormally, nor do all patients with growth deficiencies have disc displacements. It would seem that if disc displacement were a significant cause of growth deficiency, the signs and symptoms of disc displacement would be more common in this population than the normal population. The evidence does not support this, and in fact, it has been observed that the signs and symptoms do not occur more commonly

in dentofacial deformity patients.[23] Whether or not disc displacement is a cause
of growth disturbance is unclear.

Discussion

The relationship of disc displacement to pain, mandibular dysfunction,
osteoarthrosis, and growth disturbance is unclear. Alternative explanations are
plausible and should be considered. Observations during arthroscopy and
treatment outcomes after arthroscopy have provided new insights into the
pathology of temporomandibular joint internal derangement.

The role of inflammation in the temporomandibular joint was not appreciated until the use of temporomandibular joint arthroscopy. Signs of inflammation, i.e., hypervascularity and erythema, are commonly observed and have
been shown to correlate with the severity of pain.[24] Other evidence of inflammation, e.g., joint effusion, has been demonstrated with T2 weighted magnetic
resonance images.[25] Joint effusion has also been shown to be related to pain.
While disc displacement may be a cause of pain, inflammation is clearly another
cause.

Disc displacement correlates well with reciprocal clicking, but alterative
explanations exist for closed-lock. Fibrous adhesions observed during temporomandibular joint arthroscopy have been shown to be an important cause
of restricted opening.[26] Release of fibrous adhesions has restored normal range
of motion in many patients with closed-lock even when the disc has not been
repositioned. Obviously, fibrous adhesions are an alternative cause of restricted
joint movement. Other proposed causes of closed-lock include the "suction-cup
effect", the negative pressure (vacuum) effect, increased friction and low
viscosity of the synovial fluid.[13,15,16]

A relationship between disc displacement and osteoarthrosis has been
demonstrated by several authors. However, controversy exists as to whether
displacement is the cause or result of osteoarthrosis. Articular cartilage and the
underlying bone have displayed a dynamic equilibrium between changes in
form and function by tissue remodeling. The tissues will adapt to applied stress
and when the stress or loading is excessive, tissue breakdown may occur. Severe
overloading may cause irreversible changes and damage to the articular cartilage with the release of degradation products into the synovial fluid, possibly
causing synovitis. Additionally, many proteases, cytokines, growth factors, and
arachidonic acid metabolites play a role in the pathogenesis of osteoarthrosis.[27]
The causes of osteoarthrosis, although not clearly understood, are complex and
multifactorial and cannot be explained simply by disc displacement.

The evidence that disc displacement may cause growth disturbance comes
generally from small groups of temporomandibular joint patients with concomitant growth disturbances who were evaluated with various imaging.
Control groups were not included for comparison, nor were alternative explanations evaluated. The evidence that temporomandibular joint problems are no

more common within the dentofacial deformity population than the general population raises doubt as to disc derangement being a major cause of growth disturbances. As with osteoarthosis, growth disturbances probably occur as a result of many factors including genetic, trauma, pathology, and possibly disc derangement.

During the past twenty years much information has been obtained about temporomandibular joint internal derangement. Evaluation of this information indicates that the role of disc displacement as the primary pathologic factor may not be justified. Although much research remains to be done, the evidence strongly suggests that internal derangement is much more complicated than simply disc derangement. It also involves inflammation, changes in the articular cartilage, alteration in joint pressures and synovial fluid, a variety of biochemical substances, and possibly several yet to be defined factors. Consequently, the focus of classification, diagnosis, and treatment of temporomandibular joint internal derangement on disc position should be re-evaluated.

Treatment of internal derangement has been directed at procedures, both non-surgical and surgical, designed to reposition the displaced disc. Obviously, a clinician's beliefs about the importance of disc displacement determines his (her) philosophy of treatment. In view of the new evidence about temporomandibular joint internal derangement, treatment should be directed at pain management, reduction of inflammation, decreasing adverse joint loading, and restoration of normal range of motion rather than repositioning the disc.

"The evidence must ... cultivate also a sceptical state of mind toward all hypotheses – especially his own – and be ready to abandon them the moment the evidence points the other way" (Thomas Hunt Morgan)[28].

References

1 Farrar WB. Diagnosis and treatment of anterior dislocation of the articular disk. NY J Dent 1971; 41:348

2 Wilkes CH. Arthrography of the temporomandibular joint in patients with the TMJ pain-dysfunction syndrome. Minn Med 1978; 61:645

3 Farrar WB, McCarty WL. Inferior joint space arthrography and characteristics of condylar path in internal derangements of the TMJ. J Prosthet Dent 1979; 41:548

4 Katzberg RW, Dolwick MF, Bales DJ, Helms CA. Arthrotomography of the temporomandibular joint. AJR 1979; 132:949

5 McCarty WL, Farrar WB. Surgery for internal derangements of the temporomandibular joint. J Prosth Dent 1979; 42:191

6 Westesson PL, Rohlin M. Internal derangement related to osteoarthrosis in temporomandibular joint autopsy specimens. Oral Surg Oral Med Oral Pathol 1984; 57:17

7 Isberg-Holm AM, Westesson PL. Movement of disk and condyle in temporomandibular joint with clicking. An arthrographic and cineradiographic study on autopsy specimens. Acta Odontol Scand 1982; 40:151

8 Dolwick MF, Katzberg RW, Helms CA. Internal derangements of the temporomandibular joint: Fact of Fiction? J Prosthet Dent 1983; 49:415

9 Greene CS, Marbach JJ. Epidemiologic studies of mandibular dysfunction: A critical review. J Prosth Dent 1982; 48:184

10 Kaplan PA, Tu HK, Sleder PR, et al. Inferior joint space arthrography of normal TMJ: Reassessment of diagnostic criteria. Radiology 1986; 3:577

11 Kircos LT, Ortendahl DA, Mark AS, et al. Magnetic resonance imaging of the TMJ disc in asymptomatic volunteers. J Oral Maxillofac Surg 1987; 45:852

12 Kozeniauskas JJ, Ralph WJ. Bilateral arthrographic evaluation of unilateral temporomandibular joint pain and dysfunction. J Prosthet Dent 1988; 60:98

13 Sanders B. Arthroscopic surgery of the temporomandibular joint: Treatment of internal derangement with persistent closed-lock. Oral Surg Oral Med Oral Pathol 1986; 62:361

14 McCain JP. Arthroscopy of the human temporomandibular joint. J Oral Maxillofac Surg 1988; 46:648

15 Nitzan DW, Dolwick MF, Martinez A. Temporomandibular joint arthrocentesis: A simplified treatment for severe limited mouth opening. J Oral Maxillofac Surg 1991; 49:1163

16 Nitzan DW, Dolwick MF. An alternative explanation for the genesis of closed- lock symptoms in the internal derangement process. J Oral Maxillofac Surg 1991; 49:810

17 Katzberg RW, Keith DA, Buralnick WC, et al. Internal derangements and arthritis of the temporomandibular joint. Radiology 1983; 146:107

18 de Bont LGM, Liem RSB, Boering G, et al. Osteoarthritis and internal derangement of the temporomandibular joint. A light microscopic study. J Oral Maxillofac Surg 1986; 44:634

19 Hall HD, Nickerson JW. Is it time to pay more attention to disc position? J Orofacial Pain 1994; 8:90

20 Link JJ, Nickerson JW. Temporomandibular joint internal derangements in an orthognathic surgery population. Int J Orthod Orthognath Surg 1992; 7:161

21 Boering G. Temporomandibular joint arthrosis. An analysis of 400 cases. Thesis, University of Groningen, The Netherlands, 1966

22 Rickets RM. Clinical implications of the temporomandibular joint. Am J Orthod 1966; 52:416

23 Profitt WR, White RP. Surgical Orthodontic Treatment. St. Louis: Mosby Year Book, 1991, 660

24 Murakami K, Segami N, Fujimura K, et al. Correlation between pain and synovitis in patients with internal derangement of the temporomandibular joint. J Oral Maxillofac Surg 1991; 49:1159

25 Westesson PL, Brooks SL. Temporomandibular joint: Relation between MR evidence of effusion and the presence of pain and disk displacement. AJR 1992; 159:559

26 Murakami K, Segami N, Moriya Y, et al. Correlation between pain and dysfunction and intra-articular adhesions in patients with internal derangement of the temporomandibular joint. J Oral Maxillofac Surg 1992; 50:705

27 Stegenga B, de Bont LGM, Boering G, Van Willigen JD et al. Tissue responses to degenerative changes in the temporomandibular joint: a review. J Oral Maxillofac Surg 1991; 49:1079

28 Shine I, Wrobel S, Hunt Morgan T. Pioneer of Genetics, The University Press of Kentucky, Lexington, KY., 1976, p 63.

Treatment planning

Management of Temporomandibular
Joint Degenerative Diseases
ed. by B. Stegenga & L.G.M. de Bont
© 1996 Birkhäuser Verlag Basel/Switzerland

Rationale for non-surgical temporomandibular joint management

Jeffrey P. Okeson

Orofacial Pain Center; University of Kentucky, College of Dentistry, Lexington, Kentucky 40536-0084, USA

Summary: This chapter reviews the rationale for the nonsurgical management of internal derangements and osteoarthrosis. Evidence for the natural course of these disorders is presented with implications for treatment. Emphasis is placed on patient education, physical therapy, medication, and occlusal appliance therapy.

Introduction

Internal derangements refer to a group of intracapsular temporomandibular joint conditions that result from a change in the functional relationship between the mandibular condyle and the articular disc. These changes often bring about alterations in the normal sliding movements between the articular surfaces of the joint, creating certain clinical signs. In order to place this chapter into proper prospective, the clinician must keep in mind that these disorders represent only one subgroup of disorders known collectively as temporomandibular disorders. During the 1970s and 1980s, internal derangements gained enormous interest, almost to the point that other important disorders were overlooked. In reality, non-articular disorders, such as those characterized by masticatory muscle pain, are also a common source of pain and dysfunction complaints. Since the management of articular and non-articular disorders is often different, it becomes essential that the clinician is able to differentiate these two major categories of temporomandibular disorders. This process, known as diagnosis, is the most important task accomplished by the clinician. It is only through this process that appropriate therapy can be selected.

This chapter will focus on the non-surgical management of temporomandibular joint internal derangements and osteoarthrosis.

Natural course of temporomandibular joint internal derangements

The rationale for any therapy begins with a thorough understanding of the disease and its natural course. As a general rule, diseases that are progressive and destructive need to be treated quickly and aggressively. Diseases that are non-progressive and characterized by reparative processes can often be treated more palliatively and observed over time. Based on this general rule, the rationale for the management of temporomandibular arthropathies begins with an understanding of their natural course. The clinician must appreciate, however, that in the practice of dentistry the natural course of these diseases can be misinterpreted. Patients most often seek care when pain and/or dysfunction becomes great. When the clinical examination reveals signs and symptoms associated with internal derangements, the condition is easily interpreted as progressive and in need of aggressive treatment. Well-controlled, longitudinal studies are the only reliable method of evaluating the natural course of these disorders as well as the effects of therapy on the disorder's outcome. Although these studies are the most difficult to accomplish, we are most fortunate to have a few studies that shed light on these common disorders.

When studying the long-term effects of dysfunction on the temporomandibular joints, certain stages need to be identified for assessment purposes. There are three clinical stages that have been commonly used.[1] The first stage is that of reducing disc displacement. This stage is characterized by joint clicking with movement but no radiographic signs of any abnormalities in the condyle or articular eminence. The second stage is that of permanent disc displacement. This stage is characterized by a sudden restriction in mouth opening and a loss of joint sounds during movement. Radiographic changes may or may not be present during this stage depending upon the chronicity of the disorder. The third stage is that of permanent disc displacement with osseous changes as depicted by radiographic assessment. It appears that long-term studies support the concept that many patients seem to progress through these three stages.[2-7] Initially it would, therefore, appear that these disorders are progressive and need to be aggressively treated. However, when one looks carefully at these studies it is found that the final stage is not often painful or debilitating. In fact, in one longitudinal study, patients with internal derangements who were observed over thirty years were found to be no different than a control group in most evaluation parameters.[1] The greatest differences that existed between these groups were that the patients experience a slight reduction in mouth opening compared to the controls and the patients expressed a greater concern that if they opened widely the joint would hurt.[1] There was, however, no difference in the general musculoskeletal complaints of the patients and the controls in this study. Another significant difference was in the radiographic evidence of bony changes that had commonly occurred in the internal derangement group. These changes, however, were not necessarily correlated with pain nor often even with dysfunction.[2-5] This would suggest an adaptive condition resulting in a "burned-out state" with some possible residual signs (residual osteoarthrosis).

These long-term studies leave the impression that the natural course of internal derangements is towards permanent disc displacement with radiographically detectable osteoarthrotic changes. This is not always the case, however, as depicted by long-term studies that do not show consistent progression of clicking joints to permanent disc dislocation.[8-13] Therefore, long-term studies suggest that internal derangements may be progressive, but even when they are, for many patients they seem to be rather self-limiting, resulting in no significant disability.

Rationale for treatment

Understanding the natural course of these disorders allows the clinician to assume the most appropriate role as therapist. If this disorder is self-limiting for most patients, then one might question any need for aggressive therapy. Instead, the role of the therapist should be one that assists the patient through the symptomatic phase of the disorder. Palliative therapy is often the most appropriate therapy, especially in early stages of the disorder. There may, however, be some patients who will suffer greatly through this disorder and, therefore, more assistance may be needed for these patients. The aggressiveness of the therapy should only be escalated when more palliative therapy fails to control symptoms and the patient's quality of life becomes markedly decreased.

Since tissue adaptation seems to play a major role in the natural course of these disorders, treatment should be oriented towards promoting a joint condition that is most likely to repair.[14] An important part of this therapy is directed towards reducing mechanical loading of the articular surfaces.

Non-surgical treatment modalities

There are four types of therapy that should be initially considered for each patient with a symptomatic internal derangement. These therapies are patient education, physical therapy, pharmacologic therapy, and occlusal appliance therapy.

Patient education

It is very important that each patient understands the mechanism that is causing his (her) symptoms. There are several important reasons for this education. The first relates to the nature of internal derangements. Since these disorders have a significant biomechanical component, the well-informed patient can play a significant role in therapy. The patient should be instructed to decrease loading of the joint as much as possible. Softer foods, slower chewing, and smaller bites should be promoted. The patient should be told, when possible, not to allow the joint to click. The mechanics of some joints allow certain movements to occur with minimal dysfunction. When possible, these movements should be encouraged while painful movements discouraged.

Each clinician treating internal derangements should have a model or well drawn illustration of the temporomandibular joint in the office so that the patient can visualize the mechanical dysfunction. This will not only help the patient understand the condition, it also informs the patient that the disorder is common and one of which the clinician is well informed. This understanding will enhance the patient's confidence in the doctor which will likely help the patient through the adaptive phase of the disorder. The patient should also be informed of the natural course of the disorder so that reasonable expectations can be met. It is important that the patient is told that in many instances this condition is self-limiting, however the pain and dysfunction may be present for a considerable period of time. The patient should be told of the therapies that will be used and if they are not satisfactory, the clinician can offer more aggressive therapy. In the event more aggressive therapies are needed, the patient should always take part in the decision-making process. It is important that the patient realizes that the disorder is not an aggressive, tissue destructive disease such as cancer. This information will likely decrease anxiety and stress, promoting a better environment for healing.

In those patients with a permanent disc displacement, the reason for restriction in mouth opening should be shown with a model or illustration. The patient should be instructed not to attempt to force the mouth open, especially when pain is present. Instead, the patient should be told that with time, the mouth will gradually return to a more normal opening. If the patient attempts to force the mouth open too soon, tissues may be damaged and repair delayed. Once the condition has become relatively asymptomatic, the patient should then be encouraged to attempt to return back to a more normal opening as discussed in the next section.

Physical therapy

Physical therapy modalities can be helpful in managing some of the symptoms associated with internal derangements. These therapies can be divided into two broad types; those that reduce pain and those that improve function.

Physical therapy for pain reduction
In instances when pain is significant, moist heat or coolant therapy applied over the joint region can often be helpful. The clinician should suggest both heat and cold modalities to the patient since the results can be very individual. The patient should determine the most effective modality for his or her pain. Both these modalities are very conservative and can be used as often as the patient finds the need.

Thermotherapy utilizes heat as a prime mechanism and is based on the premise that heat increases circulation to the applied area. Surface heat is applied by laying a hot moist towel over the symptomatic area.[15] A hot water bottle over the towel will help maintain the heat. This combination should remain in place for 10 to 15 minutes, not to exceed 30 minutes. An electric heating pad may be used, but care must be taken not to leave it unattended.

Like thermotherapy, coolant therapy has proved to be a simple and often effective method for reducing pain. Ice should be applied directly to the symptomatic joint and/or muscles and moved in a circular motion without pressure to the tissues. The patient will initially experience an uncomfortable feeling that will quickly turn into a burning sensation. Continued icing will result in a mild aching and then numbness.[16] When numbness begins the ice should be removed. The ice should not be left on the tissues for longer than 5–7 minutes. After a period of warming a second application may be desirable. It is thought that during warming there is an increase in blood flow to the tissues assisting in tissue repair.

A common coolant therapy utilizes a vapor spray. Two of the most common sprays used are ethylchloride and fluoromethane. Vapocoolant spray is applied to the desired area for approximately five seconds. After the tissue has been rewarmed, the procedure can be repeated. Care must be taken not to allow the spray to contact the eyes, ears, nose, or mouth. A towel should be placed to protect these areas. Vapocoolant sprays do not penetrate tissue like ice and therefore it is likely that the reduction in pain is more associated with the stimulation of cutaneous nerve fibers that in turn shut down the smaller pain fibers (C fibers). This type of pain reduction is likely to be of short duration.

Two other physical therapy modalities that have been investigated are iontophoresis and cold laser. Iontophoresis is a technique by which certain medications are locally introduced into tissues. With iontophoresis the medication is placed in a pad and the pad is placed over the involved joint. Then a low electrical current is passed through the pad driving the medication into the tissue.[17] Local anesthetics and anti-inflammatory drugs are common medications used with iontophoresis.[18,19] If the medication is driven into the tissues with ultrasound, the modality is known as phonopheresis.[20]

In recent years, the cold or soft laser has been investigated for wound healing and pain relief. Presently it is not considered to be a routine physical therapy modality but is included in this section for completeness. Most studies on the cold laser report on its use in chronic musculoskeletal, rheumatic and neurological pain conditions.[21-24] It is thought that cold laser accelerates collagen synthesis, increases vascularity of healing tissues, decreases the number of micro-organisms and decreases pain. Several case studies have been published in which cold laser therapy has been used on persistent temporomandibular arthralgia.[25-27] Although the results of the studies investigating iontophoresis and cold laser have been favorable, the studies generally lack controls and adequate sample sizes. More investigations will be needed to better understand their effectiveness.

Physical therapy to improve function
Pain associated with an internal derangement or osteoarthrosis may cause the patient to restrict joint function. Although this can be helpful at first, restricting joint function can lead to chronic hypomobility and muscle atrophy. A few passive exercises can be helpful in returning the jaw to normal function. The patient should be instructed to gently open the mouth to resistance and close.

The jaw should then be moved eccentrically. Early in the process of healing these exercises should not produce any significant pain. Later, as tissue adaptation progresses, the exercises should become more active so that normal ranges of movement can be regained.

Passive distraction of a joint can increase mobility as well as inhibit the activity of muscles that pull across the joint (elevator muscles). Distraction of the temporomandibular joint is accomplished by placing the clinician's thumb in the patient's mouth over the lower second molar area on the side to be distracted. With the cranium stabilized by the other hand, the clinician places a downward force on the molar with the thumb. Distraction for relaxing muscles does not require translation of the joint but merely unloading in the closed joint position. The distraction should be maintained for several seconds and then released. It can be repeated several times. When joint mobility is the problem, distraction should be combined with manual translation of the joint.

Joint distraction has been suggested as a method of reducing a disc that has become permanently displaced.[28] Although this technique may provide some immediate success, there are only few studies that evaluate the long-term success. When managing an acute permanent disc displacement (less than a week) the technique should be attempted. If the clinician successfully reduces the disc, an anterior repositioning appliance may be indicated. Discs that have been displaced for more than several weeks are very difficult to reduce and the distraction procedure will likely fail. If the disc cannot be reduced, a centric relation appliance may be indicated merely to reduce loading forces in the joint associated with bruxing activity.

Pharmacologic therapy

Pharmacologic therapy can be an effective adjunct in managing symptoms associated with temporomandibular disorders. Patients should be aware that medication will not likely offer a solution or cure to the problem. However, medication in conjunction with appropriate physical therapy and definitive treatment does offer the most complete approach to many problems. The two most common types of medication used for internal derangements are analgesics and anti-inflammatories.

Analgesic medications
Analgesic medications can often be an important part of supportive therapy for many disorders. Control of pain is not only appreciated by the patient but it also reduces the likelihood of other complicating pain disorders such as muscle co-contraction,[29] referred pain,[30] and central sensitization.[31] The non-steroidal anti-inflammatory drugs are very helpful with most joint pains. These drugs have proven to be effective in reducing musculoskeletal pains and stop the cyclic effects of the deep pain input. There are numerous non-steroidal anti-inflammatory drugs and if one does not reduce the pain another should be tried.

Individual patients may respond differently to these medications. Continued use may result in stomach irritation so the patient should be questioned for prior stomach problems before use and monitored closely during treatment. It is suggested to take these medications with meals to lessen the likelihood of stomach irritation.

Anti-inflammatory medications

When inflammatory conditions are present (i.e., osteoarthritis), anti-inflammatories can be helpful in altering the course of the disorder. These agents suppress the body's overall response to the inflammation. Anti-inflammatory agents can be administered orally or by injection.

Oral non-steroidal anti-inflammatory drugs have already been discussed. When taken on a regular basis these medications are quite useful in the management of arthritis. It should be remembered, however, that these drugs do not immediately achieve proper blood levels and, therefore, should be taken on a regular schedule for a minimum of 2–3 weeks. The general health and condition of the patient must always be considered before these (or any) medications are prescribed; and, as is often the case, it may be necessary to consult the patient's physician regarding the advisability of such drug therapy.

Injecting an anti-inflammatory drug, such as hydrocortisone, into the joint has been advocated for the relief of pain and restricted movement.[32-36] A single intra-articular injection seems to be somewhat helpful in older patients; however, less success has been observed in patients under age 25.[34] Although a single injection is occasionally helpful, it appears that multiple injections may be harmful to the structures of the joint and should be avoided.[37,38] Therefore, the intra-articular anti-inflammatory agents should be used only in selected cases.

Occlusal appliance therapy

During the past twenty years the dental profession's attitude toward management of internal derangements has changed greatly. This is especially true with regards to the use of occlusal appliances. In the early 1970s, Farrar introduced the anterior mandibular repositioning appliance.[39] This appliance provided an occlusal relationship that required the mandible to be maintained in a forward position. The purpose of this type of appliance was an attempt to position the condyle back on the disc ("recapture the disc"). This appliance was originally suggested to be worn 24 hours a day for as long as 3–6 months. It was quickly discovered that the anterior mandibular repositioning appliance was useful in reducing painful joint symptoms.[40,41] When this appliance successfully reduced symptoms, a major treatment question was then asked: What next? Some clinicians believed that the mandible needed to be permanently maintained in this forward position. Dental procedures were suggested to create an occlusal condition that maintained the mandible in this therapeutic relationship. Accomplishing this task was never a simple dental procedure. Others felt that once the discal ligaments repaired, the mandible should be returned to its normal position in the fossa (step the mandible back to its musculoskeletally stable position) and the disc would still remain in proper position (recaptured). Although one approach was more conservative than the other, neither has been supported by long-term data.

In early shortterm studies, the anterior repositioning appliance proved to be much more effective in reducing joint symptoms than the more traditional centric relation appliance.[13,40,42-46] This, of course, lead the profession to believe that returning the disc to its proper relationship with the condyle was an essential part of the treatment. The greatest insight regarding the appropriateness of a treatment modality, however, is gained from long-term studies. Forty patients with various internal derangements were evaluated 2.5 years after anterior repositioning therapy and a stepback procedure.[13] No patients received any occlusal alterations. It was reported that 66% of the patients still had joint sounds, but only 25% were still experiencing pain problems. If the criteria for success in this study were the elimination of both pain and joint sounds, then success was achieved in only 28%. Other long-term studies have reported similar findings.[11,46] If the presence of asymptomatic joint sounds is not a criterion for failure, however, then the success rate for anterior repositioning appliances rises to 75%. The issue that must be addressed, therefore, is the clinical significance of asymptomatic joint sounds. Joint sounds are very common in the general population. In many cases it appears that they are not related to pain or decreased joint mobility.[47,48] If all clicking joints always progressed to more serious conditions, then this would be a good indication to treat each and every joint that clicked. The presence of unchanging joint sounds over time, however, indicates that the structures involved can adapt to less than optimum functional relationships.[49] The fact that clicking sounds persist over time does not necessarily indicate a progressive disorder. Long-term studies do, however, give insight as to how the joint responds to anterior repositioning therapy. In many patients, advancing the mandible forward for a time prevents the condyle from articulating with the highly vascularized, well innervated, retrodiscal tissues. This is the likely explanation for an almost immediate reduction of intracapsular pain. During the forward repositioning the retrodiscal tissues undergo adaptive and reparative changes.[50] These tissues can become fibrotic and avascular.[51-58]

We know now that discs are not generally recaptured by anterior repositioning appliances.[59] Instead, as the condyle returns to the fossa it moves posteriorly to articulate on the adapted retrodiscal tissues. If these tissues have adequately adapted, loading occurs without pain. The condyle now functions on the newly adapted retrodiscal tissues although the disc is still anteriorly displaced. The result is a painless joint that may continue to click with condylar movement. At one time the dental profession believed that the presence of joint sounds indicated treatment failure. Long-term follow-up studies have given the profession new insight regarding success and failure. We, like our orthopedic colleagues, have learned to accept that some dysfunction is likely to persist once joint structures have been altered. Controlling pain, while allowing joint structures to adapt, appears to be the most important role of the therapist.

It should be noted that a few long-term studies do support the concept that permanent alteration of the occlusal condition can be successful in controlling most major symptoms.[45,60] This treatment, however, requires extensive dental therapy and one must question the need when natural adaptation appears to work well for most patients. Reconstruction of the dentition or orthodontic therapy should be reserved only for those patients who present with a significant orthopedic instability.

The use of anterior repositioning appliance therapy is not without adverse consequences. A certain percentage of patients who wear these appliances develop a posterior open-bite. This may be the result of a reversible, myostatic contracture of the inferior lateral pterygoid muscle. When this condition exists, a gradual relengthening of the muscle can be accomplished by slowly stepping the condyle back to the more stable anterosuperior position in the fossa. This can be accomplished by slowly adjusting the appliance to allow the condyle to return to the musculoskeletally stable position, by slowly decreasing use of the appliance, or both. The degree of myostatic contracture that develops is likely to be proportional to the length of time the appliance has been worn. As already mentioned, when these appliances were first introduced, they were suggested to be worn 24 hours a day for 3 to 6 months. The philosophy now is to reduce the wearing time as much as possible so as to limit the adverse effects on the occlusion. For many patients, full-time use is not necessary to reduce symptoms. When possible, the patient should wear the appliance only at night to protect the retrodiscal tissues from heavy loading (bruxism). If the symptoms can be controlled without wearing the appliance during the day, the development of myostatic contracture will be avoided.

For some patients with an internal derangement a more traditional muscle relaxation (centric relation) appliance can reduce symptoms. This is the appliance of choice since the risk of altering the occlusion is minimized. It should also be noted that both appliances should provide full arch coverage so as to avoid tooth eruption. If symptoms persist with only night-time use of the appliance, the patient may need to wear it more often. Day-time use may be necessary for a few weeks. As soon as the patient becomes symptom-free, the use of the appliance should be gradually reduced. If reduction of use creates a return of symptoms, either there has not been adequate time for tissue repair or significant orthopedic instability is present. In most cases, it is best to assume that inadequate time for tissue repair is the reason for return of symptoms. The anterior repositioning appliance should therefore be reinstituted and more time given for tissue repair. When repeated attempts to eliminate the appliance fail to control symptoms, orthopedic instability should be suspected. When this occurs, the appliance should be gradually reduced allowing the condyle to return to the musculoskeletally stable (superior anterior) position. Once the condyles are in this position, the occlusal condition should be assessed for orthopedic stability. Orthopedic instability is not a common finding but when it is present, dental therapy may be indicated.

If the disc is permanently displaced, an anterior repositioning appliance is contra-indicated. This type of appliance will likely aggravate the anteriorly positioned disc. Patient education, physical therapy and medications are the best methods for promoting adaptation of the permanently displaced disc. If the patient is suspected to have significant bruxism, a muscle relaxation or flat plane appliance is indicated to reduce loading of the retrodiscal tissues during sleep. A lack of adaptation is usually accompanied by pain.

Conclusion

Significant evidence exists to support the concept that non-surgical therapies are important treatment options for temporomandibular arthropathies. Non-surgical therapies are likely to assist in symptom relief and tissue adaptation and therefore should be the first avenue of management. Surgical therapies should be considered only when non-surgical efforts fail to adequately reduce symptoms over a reasonable period of time, and the patient's quality of life is being significantly affected.

References

1   de Leeuw R, Boering G, Stegenga B, de Bont LGM. Temporomandibular joint osteoarthrosis: clinical and radiographic characteristics 30 years after non-surgical treatment: a preliminary report. J Craniomandibular Pract 1993; 11:15
2   Boering G. Arthrosis deformans van het kaakgewricht. Thesis, University of Groningen, The Netherlands, 1966
3   Boering G, Stegenga B, de Bont LGM. Temporomandibular joint osteoarthritis and internal derangement. Part I: Clinical course and initial treatment. Int Dent J 1990; 40:339
4   Rasmussen OC. Clinical findings during the course of temporomandibular arthropathy. Scand J Dent Res 1981; 89:283
5   Rasmussen OC. Temporomandibular arthropathy. Int J Oral Surg 1983; 12:365
6   Stegenga B, de Bont LGM, Boering G. Osteoarthrosis as the cause of craniomandibular pain and dysfunction: a unifying concept. J Oral Maxillofac Surg 1989; 47:249
7   Nickerson JW, Boering G. Natural course of osteoarthrosis as it relates to internal derangements of the temporomandibular joint. Oral Maxillofac Surg Clin North Am 1989; 1:27
8   Bush FM, Carter WH. TMJ clicking and facial pain, J Dent Res 1983; 62:304, abstr. 1217
9   Greene CS, Turner C, Laskin D. Long-term outcome of TMJ clicking in 100 MPD patients. J Dent Res 1982; 61:218, abstr. 359
10 Greene CS, Laskin D. Long-term status of TMJ clicking in patients with myofascial pain and dysfunction. J Am Dent Assoc 1988; 117:461
11 Lundh H, Westesson PL, Kopp S. A three-year follow-up of patients with reciprocal temporomandibular joint clicking. Oral Surg Oral Med Oral Pathol 1987; 63:530
12 Magnusson T, Egermark-Ericksson I, Carlsson GE. Five-year longitudinal study of signs and symptoms of mandibular dysfunction in adolescents. J Craniomandibular Pract 1986, 4:339
13 Okeson JP. The long-term treatment of disc-interference disorders. J Prosthet Dent 1988; 60:611
14 de Leeuw R, Boering G, Stegenga B, de Bont LGM. TMJ osteoarthrosis and internal derangement 30 years after non-surgical treatment. J Orofacial Pain 1994; 8:18

15 Nelson SJ, Ash MM. An evaluation of a moist heat pad for the treatment of TMJ/muscle pain dysfunction. J Craniomandibular Pract 1988; 6:355

16 Satlerthwaite JR. Ice massage. Pain Mgt 1989; 2:116

17 Lark MR, Gangarosa LP. Iontophoresis: an effective modality for the treatment of inflammatory disorders of the temporomandibular joint and myofascial pain. J Craniomandibular Pract 1990; 8:108

18 Gangarosa LP. Iontophoresis in Dental Practice. Chicago: Quintessence Publ, 1983

19 Gangarosa LP, Ikeshima A, Morihana T, et al. Ionotophoresis (IONTO) of lidocaine (Lido) into the TMJ of rabbits. J Dent Res 1991; 70:444, abstr. 1428

20 Kleinkort JA, Wood F. Phonopheresis with one percent versus ten percent hydrocortisone. Phys Ther 1985; 55:1320

21 Kleinkort JA, Foley R. Laser acupuncture. Its use in physical therapy. Am J Acupuncture 1984; 12:51

22 SynderMackler L, Bork CE. Effect of heliumneon laser irradiation on peripheral sensory nerve latency. Phys Ther 1988; 68:223

23 Walker J. Relief from chronic pain from low-power laser irradiation. Neurosci Lett 1983; 43:339

24 Bliddal H, Hellesen C, Ditleusen P, et al. Soft laser therapy of rheumatoid arthritis. Scand J Rheumatol 1987; 16:225

25 Hansson TL. Infrared laser in the treatment of craniomandibular arthrogenenous pain. J Prosthet Dent 1989; 61:614

26 Palano D, Martelli M. A clinic statistical investigation of laser effect in the treatment of pain and dysfunction of the temporomandibular joint (TMJ). Med Laser Report 1985; 2:21

27 Bezuur NJ, Habets LLMH, Hansson TL. The effect of therapeutic laser treatment in patients with craniomandibular disorders. J Craniomandib Disord Facial Oral Pain 1988; 2:83

28 Okeson JP. Management of temporomandibular disorders and occlusion, 3rd ed. St. Louis: Mosby Year Book, 1993; 413

29 Okeson JP. Management of temporomandibular disorders and occlusion, 3rd ed. St. Louis: Mosby Year Book, 1993; 182

30 Bell WE. Orofacial Pains: classification, diagnosis, and management. 4th ed. Chicago: Year Book Med Publishers, 1989; 67

31 Woolf CJ, Thompson SWN. The induction and maintenance of central sensitization is dependent on N-methyl-D-aspartic acid receptor activation: implications for the treatment of post-injury pain hypersensitivity. Pain 1991; 44:293

32 Henny FA. Intraarticular injection of hydrocortisone into the temporomandibular joint. J Oral Surg 1954; 12:314

33 Toller PA. Osteoarthritis of the mandibular condyle. Br Dent J 1973; 134:233

34 Toller PA. Non-surgical treatment of dysfunctions of the temporomandibular joint. Oral Sci Rev 1976; 7:70

35 Kopp S. Long-term effects of intra-articular injections of sodium hyaluronate and corticosteroids on temporomandibular joint arthritis. J Oral Maxillofac Surg 1987; 45:929

36 Wenneberg B, Kopp S, Grondahl, HG. Long-term effect of intra-articular injections of a glucocorticosteroid into the TMJ: a clinical and radiographic 8-year followup. J Craniomandib Disord Facial Pain 1991; 5:11

37 Poswillo DE: Experimental investigation of the effects of intra-articular hydrocortisone and high condylectomy on the mandibular condyle. Oral Surg 1970; 30:161

38 Zarb GA, Speck JE. The treatment of mandibular dysfunction. In Temporomandibular joint: function and dysfunction. Zarb GA, Carlsson GE (eds). St Louis: Mosby, 1979

39 Farrar WB. Differentiation of temporomandibular joint dysfunction to simplify treatment. J Prosthet Dent 1972; 28:629

40 Anderson GC, Schulte JK, Goodkind RJ. Comparative study of two treatment methods for internal derangements of the temporomandibular joint. J Prosthet Dent 1985; 53:392

41 Gazit E, Lieberman M, Eini R, et al. Prevalence of functional disturbances in 10–18 year old Israeli school children. J Oral Rehabil 1984; 11:307

42 Burns R, McKinney J, Chase D, Anderson D. Occlusal splint therapy for treatment of internal derangements: retrospective study. J Dent Res 1983; 62:304, abstr. 1215

43 Lundh H, Westesson PL, Kopp S, et al. Anterior repositioning splint in the treatment of temporomandibular joints with reciprocal clicking: Comparison with a flat occlusal splint and an untreated control group. Oral Surg Oral Med Oral Pathol 1985; 60:131

44 Lundh H, et al. Diskrepositioning onlays in the treatment of temporomandibular joint disk

displacement: Comparison with a flat occlusal splint and with no treatment. Oral Surg Oral Med Oral Pathol 1988; 66:155

45   McGowan P, McKinney J, Chase D, Anderson D. Treatment of anterior disc displacement with Jankelson Myosplint: retrospective study. J Dent Res 1983; 62:304, abstr. 1216

46   Moloney F, Howard JA. Internal derangement of the temporomandibular joint. III. Anterior repositioning splint therapy. Aust Dent J 1986; 31:1

47   Heikinheimo K, Salmi K, Myllarniemi S, Kirveskari P. Symptoms of craniomandibular disorders in a sample of Finnish adolescents at the ages of 12 and 15 years. Eur J Orthod 1989; 11:325

48   Vincent SD, Lilly GE. Incidence and characterization of temporomandibular joint sounds in adults, J Am Dent Assoc 1988; 116:203

49   Stegenga B, de Bont LGM, Boering G, van Willigen JD. Tissue responses to degenerative changes in the temporomandibular joint. J Oral Maxillofac Surg 1991; 49:1079

50   Bay R, Timmis D. Histopathology of human TMJ disc perforation after anterior repositioning splint therapy. J Dent Res 1989; 68:1004, abstr. 1096

51   Akerman S, Kopp S, Rohlin M. Histological changes in temporomandibular joints from elderly individuals, Acta Odontol Scand 1986; 44:231

52   Baldioceda F, Bibb C, Pullinger A. Morphologic variability in the human TMJ disc and posterior attachment. J Dent Res 1989; 68:229, abstr. 384

53   Blaustein DI, Scapino RP. Remodeling of the temporomandibular joint disk and posterior attachment in disk displacement specimens in relation to glycosaminoglycan content. Plastic Recon Surg 1986; 78:19

54   Hall MB, Brown RW, Baughman RA. Histologic appearance of the bilaminar zone in internal derangement of the temporomandibular joint. Oral Surg Oral Med Oral Pathol 1984; 58:375

55   Salo L, Raustia A, Pernu H, Virtanen K. Internal derangement of the temporomandibular joint: a histochemical study. J Oral Maxillofac Surg 1991; 49:171

56   Scapino RP. Histopathology associated with malposition of the human temporomandibular joint disc. Oral Surg Oral Med Oral Pathol 1983; 55:382

57   Solberg WK, Hansson TL, Nordstrom B. The temporomandibular joint in young adults at autopsy: a morphologic classification and evaluation. J Oral Rehabil 1985; 12:303

58   Solberg WK, Bibb CA, Nordstrom BB, Hansson TL. Malocclusion associated with temporomandibular joint changes in young adults of autopsy. Am J Orthod 1986; 89:326

59   Kirk WS. Magnetic resonance imaging and tomographic evaluation of occlusal appliance treatment for advanced internal derangement of the temporomandibular joint. J Oral Maxillofac Surg 1991; 49:9

60   Tallents RH, Katzberg RW, Macher DJ, Roberts CA. Use of protrusive splint therapy in anterior disk displacement of the temporomandibular joint: A 1 to 3 year follow-up. J Prosthet Dent 1990; 63:336

Management of Temporomandibular
Joint Degenerative Diseases
ed. by B. Stegenga & L.G.M. de Bont
© 1996 Birkhäuser Verlag Basel/Switzerland

Rationale for surgical temporomandibular joint management

Rudolf H. Reich

*Department of Oral and Maxillofacial Surgery, Rheinische Friedrich-Wilhelms University,
D-53111 Bonn, Germany*

Summary: Surgery is indicated when certain requirements and prerequisites are met, and these are addressed in this chapter. For internal derangements at different stages as well as osteoarthrosis, a therapeutic spectrum is available, including arthrocentesis, arthroscopic lysis and lavage, refined arthroscopic surgery, and open joint surgical methods. Arthroscopy is the first modality of choice for surgical treatment because it combines the possibility of exact disorder staging with a therapeutic effect in a considerable number of patients.

Introduction

When compared with extremity joint surgery, it seems peculiar that temporo-mandibular joint surgery for osteoarthrosis and internal derangement is still controversial. Current controversies include indications for surgery and surgical techniques. The question of indication for surgery in certain temporo-mandibular arthropathies, such as internal derangement and osteoarthrosis, seems to be related to historical factors. Surgical procedures that were carried out on a routine basis in the 1940s and 1950s were abandoned by several investigators because of complications such as continuing or increased post-operative pain, recurrence of osteoarthrosis, ankylosis, or facial paralysis.[1,2,3] In retrospect, poor patient selection may have been responsible for these failures. In addition, it must be appreciated that fewer surgical options were available in the past.

Functional surgery for temporomandibular joint degenerative diseases should be based on proper patient selection and treatment concepts. Long-term studies have shown that a non-surgical approach can lead to good results in terms of pain reduction and function improvement,[4] and this should be considered when establishing indications for surgery and informed consent. Nevertheless, frequently patients wish to have their pain and/or dysfunction relieved as quickly as possible, even when surgery is necessary to achieve this.

Basic considerations related to surgical treatment

Modern approaches to treatment of temporomandibular joint problems include arthrography, computerized tomography, and magnetic resonance imaging, which has almost replaced arthrography. Arthroscopy has made it possible to begin to stage the disease, and consequently, surgical therapy can be planned and performed more precisely.

Diagnosis, treatment planning, and post-operative management are performed in a multidisciplinary way, e.g., in co-operation with a prosthodontist or physical therapist. Information from other fields, such as psychology, influences treatment planning as well. For instance, several forms of muscular hyperactivity are frequently connected with a lack of stress control,[5] and patients showing signs of muscular hyperactivity do not tend to respond very well to surgical temporomandibular joint therapy.[6]

Improvements in surgical approaches are evident in the availability of specially designed instruments and refined techniques such as the postauricular approach.[7] Saving the facial nerve does not seem to be a problem anymore.[8] The possibilities of arthroscopic surgery are further examples of the progress made in surgical techniques during recent years.

As far as indication criteria for surgical interventions are concerned, the borderline between non-surgical and surgical therapy demands particular attention. How and for how long should nonsurgical therapy be persued before surgery is considered? Are there any cases in which surgery is the only rational treatment option? The introduction of arthroscopy and, more recently, arthrocentesis have widened our surgical scope considerably.[9] Yet, these innovations have brought about the necessity to decide between these methods and open surgery. Moreover, the proper surgical procedure for a given disorder is a constant subject of discussion. In what stages of temporomandibular joint degenerative disease is soft tissue surgery or arthroscopic surgery indicated, and what kind of treatment is recommended for manifest osteoarthrosis?

Osteoarthrosis: pathophysiologic considerations

Before trying to answer these questions, some features about the pathophysiology of osteoarthrosis must be addressed. Osteoarthrosis appears to represent a dynamic process. Changes in the subchondral bone of the mandibular condyle aggravate the process of degenerative destruction.[10] On the other hand, an earlier supposed "natural history", which postulated an inevitable course from reducing disc displacement to osteoarthrosis,[11] obviously does not generally apply. Degenerative changes may arrest at any stage. Osteoarthrotic changes of the temporomandibular joint can stop and become asymptomatic under favorable circumstances by adaptation.

Two basic types of osteoarthrosis have been identified.[12] In type 1 osteoarthrosis, degenerative changes of the condyle and/or the articular eminence affect the joint in a period of 9-16 months. Either spontaneously or with non-surgical therapy the process gradually "burns out" within this period of time. The improvement of symptoms corresponds with subsequent flattening of the condylar head. It ends up in a "gliding joint without a disc".[13] A question in the literature is whether this entity really represents osteoarthrosis or whether it should be considered a form of progressive remodeling with symptoms. The other type (type 2 osteoarthrosis) can be observed at any age in adults and is progressive in terms of signs and symptoms. Even after 12–16 months of observation there is no improvement, and it is most probable that clinical recovery does not occur spontaneously. Thus, in the case of degenerative changes in hard tissues, it seems reasonable to observe for at least 9–12 months before considering surgery, since in this phase the two types of osteoarthrosis cannot be distinguished one from the another. Nonsurgical therapy, i.e., observation alone, occlusal or physical treatment, can be performed during this phase. Only when there is no trend toward improvement should surgery be considered. In all other cases of internal derangement and osteoarthrosis, at least one adequate trial of nonsurgical treatment should be performed before considering surgery.

Indication criteria for surgery

The following criteria for surgical treatment seem to be accepted by the majority of surgeons:

- presence of pain and/or impairment of function
- evidence of morphologic changes
- high probability of a causal relationship between signs and symptoms and morphologic changes
- adequate non-surgical treatment appears ineffective
- absence of contra-indications
- probability of improvement by surgery
- post-operative interdisciplinary therapy possible
- good patient compliance

All of these criteria must be met for each individual case.

The surgical treatment itself should be based on pathophysiology as much as possible. For Wilkes' stage III internal derangement,[14] arthroscopic lysis and lavage has been shown to be a valid procedure. In some centers, more refined techniques such as arthroscopic anterior release in combination with scarring of the retrodiscal tissue have been performed successfully. In closed-lock cases, these procedures concur with arthrocentesis. However, long-term results of this technique are not yet available. For symptomatic disc perforations, shaving procedures have been performed arthroscopically with success. The options for open surgery for these disorders and for disc dislocation include disc repositioning, discoplasty, and discectomy with or without interposition. Most probably, the good functional results obtained with these modalities are due to anatomical reconstruction as well as to the adaptative changes induced.[15]

A biologic system, like the temporomandibular joint, is not characterized by static behaviour but by a continuously changing balance between detrimental influences and adaptation. The goal of surgery should be to help to improve the joint's structural features in order to enhance adaptation, keeping in mind that any surgical treatment creates adverse effects as well. For example, in progressive osteoarthrosis, direct contact between the condyle and the articular eminence seems to be an irritating factor that prevents adaptation. Thus, it seems reasonable to create space within the joint cavity, taking away perpetuating changes in the subchondral area, and making it possible for undifferentiated mesenchymal cells to provide for a new covering for the condylar surface.

From the experience of the past 15 years, we know that hyperactivity of the jaw muscles may be an important cause of unfavorable results following temporomandibular joint surgery. Muscular hyperactivity shows itself in various guises.[16] Several simple clinical symptoms should be a warning in terms of indication for surgery:

– pain outside the region of the temporomandibular joint
– pain at rest
– bilateral occurrence of symptoms
– changing location of symptoms
– symptoms present for more than four years
– previous surgery.

In high degree muscular hyperactivity surgery can even be contra-indicated. Although scientific data about severe forms of muscular hyperactivity are lacking, we can assume that neurologic phenomena play a significance role. For example, patients with Meige's syndrome, a rare disorder, show very painful attacks of jaw muscle spasm that can lead to progressive osteoarthrotic changes in the temporomandibular joints. Only when the muscular hyperfunction is minimized over time by adequate neurologic treatment can surgery be considered.

Patients with symptoms of less than four years' duration who show no signs of muscular hyperactivity, localized pain in the temporomandibular joint associated with function, or unilateral symptoms can be expected to respond to surgery in a more predictable way.

Objectives of surgery

The objectives for temporomandibular joint surgery should be realistic. In general, the main objectives include:

– elimination of pain
– improvement of function
– enhancement of adaptation
– cessation of disease progression

Complications

With today's methods, the rate of surgical complications is very low. In our own experience of 324 consecutive patients (358 surgeries) treated between 1983 and 1993 by arthrotomy, an overall complications rate of 2.7% was seen. This included permanent weakness of the frontal ramus of the facial nerve (0.7%) and bite changes (1.1%). These numbers are consistent with the literature. Thus, complications are not a restrictive factor for surgical treatment of temporomandibular joint osteoarthrosis.

Sequencing of surgical procedures

After the decision to operate has been made based on the considerations stated above, sequencing of surgical procedures comes into focus. For internal derangements, arthroscopic inspection as well as lysis and lavage should be the first step. Some authors advocate arthrocentesis as a first procedure, particularly for patients with a relatively recent permanent disc displacement presenting with locking. Arthroscopic anterior release and scarring of the retrodiscal tissue may be a future option in later stages of disc displacement. In cases showing persisting symptoms following these procedures, open disc repositioning would be the next option.

Symptomatic small perforations of the retrodiscal tissue can be improved by arthroscopic shaving. A discoplasty, however, appears to be one of the most effective treatment modalities in open surgery.

For patients with a large perforation, again, arthroscopic shaving can be the first option. Yet, so far, long-term results of this procedure are inconclusive. As an open procedure, discectomy or discectomy in combination with a high condylectomy with or without interposition of alloplastic or biologic material has been described as being effective.

For patients showing bony changes on the radiograph, arthroscopic procedures are still debatable because of a lack of scientific data so far. Following convention, interpositional arthroplasty or pure arthroplasty would be called for. Yet in interpositional arthroplasty, the type of interposition as well as the question of permanent or temporary implantation are currently under discussion. It must be emphasized that in cases of morphologic changes of the bony structures of the temporomandibular joint, open soft tissue surgery alone obviously has limited effectiveness. Some reports in the literature propose condylotomy as an alternative for arthroplasty or interpositional arthroplasty.

Condylectomy and autologous or even alloplastic reconstruction of the temporomandibular joint should only be considered in very rare cases of recurrent progressive osteoarthrosis following previous surgical treatments as well as in cases of early ankylosis.

It should be emphasized that this sequencing of treatment is not yet backed by extensive scientific data. In the future, the outcome of open surgery could get worse following the proposed sequencing concept because the "winners" have been treated by arthrocentesis and arthroscopic procedures. Earlier stages of the disease seem to respond better to surgical treatment anyhow.

Summary

It has been shown that the majority of patients presenting with various stages of temporomandibular joint osteoarthrosis improve with time, with or without non-surgical therapy. Consequently, surgery is indicated only when specific requirements are fulfilled and prerequisites are met.

For disc dislocation at different stages as well as osteoarthrosis, a therapeutic spectrum including arthrocentesis, arthroscopic lysis and lavage, arthroscopic surgery, and open joint surgical methods is available. Arthroscopy is the first modality of choice for surgical treatment because for many patients it combines the possibility of exact disease staging with a therapeutic effect.

References

1 Wassmund M. Zur Chirurgie des Kiefergelenkes. Zahn, Mund u. Kieferheilk in Vorträgen 1951; 6:68
2 Trauner R. Diskussionsbemerkungen. In: Fortschritte der Kiefer und Gesichtschirurgie, Bd. VI. Schuchardt, K (ed). Stuttgart: Thieme, 1960; 327
3 Reichenbach E, Grimm G. Indikation und Prognose der Diskusexzision. In: Fortschritte der Kiefer und Gesichtschirurgie. Bd. VI. Schuchardt, K (ed). Stuttgart: Thieme, 1960; 130
4 de Leeuw R, Boering G, Stegenga B, de Bont LGM. Temporomandibular joint osteoarthrosis: clinical and radiographic characters 30 years after nonsurgical treatment. A preliminary report. J Craniomandibular Pract 1993; 11:15
5 Rugh JD. Psychological factors in the etiology of masticatory pain and dysfunction. In: The presidents' conference of the etiology, diagnosis and treatment of TMJ disorders. Laskin DM et al. (eds). Chicago: Am Dent Assoc Publ, 1983; 85
6 Reich RH, Bothe KJ. Der Schmerz als Indikation für die funktionelle Kiefergelenkchirurgie. Deutsche Zahnarztl Z 1990; 45:55
7 Reich RH, Bothe KJ. Zur Wahl des Zugangsweges zum Kiefergelenk aus esthetischer Sicht. Dtsch Z Mund Kiefer Gesichts Chir 1990; 14:67
8 Al Kayat A, Bramley P. A modified preauricular approach to the temporomandibular joint and malar arch. Br J Oral Maxillofac Surg 1979; 17:91
9 Nitzan DW, Dolwick MF, Martinez GA. Temporomandibular joint arthrocentesis. J Oral Maxillofac Surg 1991; 49:1163
10 de Bont LGM, Boering G, Liem RSB, Eulderink F, Westesson PL. Osteoarthritis and internal derangement of the temporomandibular joint: a lightmicroscopic study. J Oral Maxillofac Surg 1986; 44:634
11 Ireland VE. The problem of the "clicking jaw". Proc Roy Soc Med 1951; 44:191
12 Laskin DM. Surgery of the temporomandibular joint. In: Temporomandibular joint problems. Biologic diagnosis and treatment. Solberg WK, Clark GT (eds). Chicago: Quintessence, 1980; 111
13 Steinhardt G. Zur Pathologie und Therapie des Kiefergelenkknackens. Dtsch Z Chir 1933; 241:531
14 Wilkes CH. Internal derangement of the temporomandibular joint: pathologic variations. Arch Otolaryng Head Neck Surg 1989; 115:469
15 Westesson PL, Cohen JM, Tallents RH. Magnetic resonance imaging of temporomandibular joint after surgical treatment of internal derangement. Oral Surg Oral Med Oral Pathol 1991; 71:407
16 Reich RH, Rossbach E. Erscheinungsformen muskulärer Hyperaktivität im Kiefer und Gesichtsbereich – ein Beitrag zur Differentialdiagnose und Therapie von Kiefergelenkerkrankungen. Dtsch Zahnarztl Z 1988; 43:11

Management of Temporomandibular
Joint Degenerative Diseases
ed. by B. Stegenga & L.G.M. de Bont
© 1996 Birkhäuser Verlag Basel/Switzerland

Orthognathic considerations in temporomandibular joint treatment planning

D. Bram Tuinzing

Department of Oral and Maxillofacial Surgery/Oral Pathology, University Hospital VU/ACTA, 1007 MB Amsterdam, The Netherlands

Summary: Basically, five groups of dentofacial deformity can be distinguished. The behaviour of the temporomandibular joint after orthognathic surgery in each of these groups is discussed in this chapter. Recommendations for temporomandibular joint management in relation to the surgical correction of dentofacial deformities are provided.

Introduction

Temporomandibular joint functioning is influenced when corrections of dentofacial deformities are carried out. To remain within functional limits, the joints must adjust structurally during the period when the dental arches are aligned orthodontically, as well as after orthognathic surgery.

Based on the considerable experience obtained at the Department of Oral and Maxillofacial Surgery of the Free University of Amsterdam, a classification of five groups of dentofacial deformities has been developed.[1] Each group has its own treatment approach and implications with regard to the temporomandibular joint after surgical intervention.[2]

Classification of dentofacial deformities

The majority of dentofacial deformities can be classified in one of the following groups:[1]

- mandibular prognathism
- mandibular prognathism with open bite
- mandibular retrognathism with low/normal mandibular plane angle
- relative mandibular retrognathism
- absolute mandibular retrognathism with high mandibular plane angle.

The terms used to designate these groups might give the impression that only deformities in the mandible are included. However, the terms must be considered as 'names of the game'. For example, the reversed incisal relationship in mandibular prognathism might be due to maxillary retrognathism, alveolar mandibular prognathism, pseudoprognathism, maxillary hypoplasia, etc. Similarly, a class II malocclusion might be the result of mandibular retrognathism as well as of maxillary prognathism. For each group a specific approach can be defined in terms of a set of rules, which refer to stability,[3] psychosocial aspects,[4] and temporomandibular joint behaviour.

Mandibular prognathism without open bite

This deformity is characterized by a reversed overjet (figure 1A). After orthodontic treatment, aiming at coincidental and regular dental arches, correction can be carried out by setback of the mandible, advancement of the maxilla, or a clockwise rotational movement of the bimaxillary complex. The stability of any of these treatment modatilities appears to be satisfactory.

Regarding the psychosocial aspects, the considerable change in facial appearance might cause emotional problems as the 'old' compensating mechanisms are not in concordance with the 'new' face.

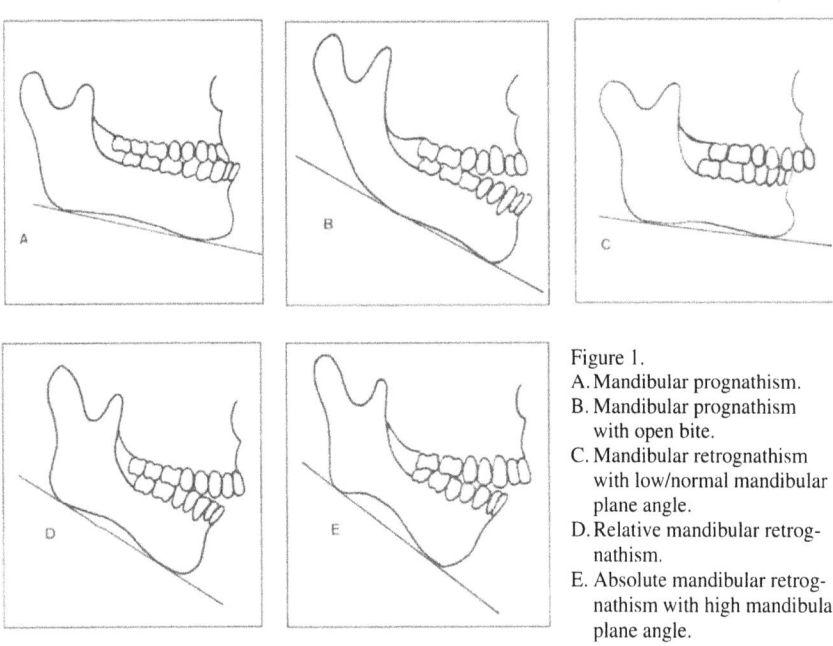

Figure 1.
A. Mandibular prognathism.
B. Mandibular prognathism with open bite.
C. Mandibular retrognathism with low/normal mandibular plane angle.
D. Relative mandibular retrognathism.
E. Absolute mandibular retrognathism with high mandibular plane angle.

Mandibular prognathism with open bite

This deformity is characterized by a reversed overjet and an open bite (figure 1B), and thus includes both vertical and horizontal components. After orthodontic treatment, aiming at well-aligned dental arches, the vertical component is best corrected by a le Fort I osteotomy. The resulting increase in the horizontal component caused by autorotation of the mandible can then be corrected by a mandibular setback. The skeletal stability of this bimaxillary intervention appears to be satisfactory, although the anterior open bite may recur due to relapse of the anterior teeth in the transversal plane, possibly due to insufficient adaptation of the tongue.

The psychosocial aspects are comparable to those of the mandibular prognathism without open bite.

Mandibular retrognathism with low/normal mandibular plane angle

This deformity is characterized by an increased overjet (figure 1C). Although this overjet might be due to a maxillary prognathism, it is felt that surgical posterior replacement of the maxilla leads to disappointing results from an esthetic point of view. As a result, this technique has become more or less redundant.

Depending on the position of the chin, the curve of Spee is more or less leveled before surgical advancement of the mandible is carried out. Occasionally, bimaxillary surgery is necessary either to control the position of the chin, to prevent the occurrence of a 'squarelike' face, or to prevent unstable anticlockwise advancement of the mandible. The stability of these treatment modalities appears to be satisfactory.

From a psychosocial point of view some difficulties might occur in the pre-surgical orthodontic phases as the orthodontic appliance attracts attention to the 'compensated' deformity.

Relative and absolute mandibular retrognathism with high mandibular plane angle

Relative and absolute mandibular retrognathism differ mainly with regard to the need for mandibular advancement in the latter. With relative mandibular retrognathism (figure 1D), the mandible is considered of normal size and retruded secondary to a vertical maxillary hyperplasia. Thus, posterior impaction of the maxilla leads to correction of the mandibular deformity by anticlockwise autorotation of the mandible. Treating absolute mandibular retrognathism (figure 1E), this way however, results in a setback of the maxilla, which has a negative influence on the esthetics of the face as mentioned above. Therefore, bimaxillary surgery, i.e., advancement of the mandible and posterior impaction of the maxilla to prevent undesired anticlockwise rotational movement of the mandible, are indicated. Stability in relative mandibular retrognathism cases appears to be very good, while in the absolute mandibular retrognathism group relapse might occur due to changes in the volume of the condyles.

Because the desire for esthetic improvement plays a major role in both groups, and because the outcome of surgery for absolute mandibular retrognathism may be unstable, pre-surgical psychological evaluation is strongly recommended.

Interrelationship between the temporomandibular joint and dentofacial deformity

Temporomandibular joint complaints sometimes be the reason for carrying out orthognathic surgery, as malocclusion may in some instances lead to jaw displacement and subsequent temporomandibular joint problems. Conversely, orthognathic surgery, which occasionally involves intermaxillary fixation or a 'forced position' of the condyles due to plate and screw fixation, may give rise to temporomandibular problems.[5,6]

Anatomical aspects of the temporomandibular joint

The depth of the articular fossa and the angle of the posterior slope of the articular eminence are important when considering orthognathic surgery. Compared with patients without dysfunction, patients with articular eminence show an anterior disc displacement that is much steeper on average (figure 2).[7]

Figure 2.
Steepness of articular eminence in patients without temporomandibular joint dysfunction as compared with patients with an anterior disc displacement.

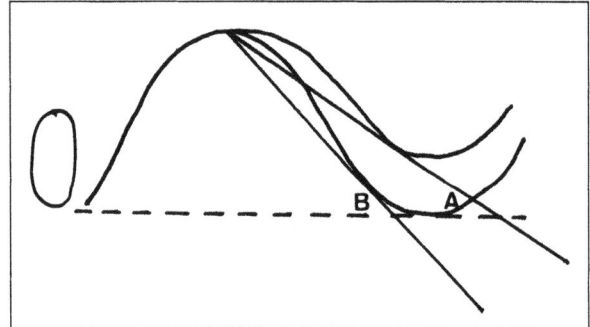

When patients with mandibular retrognathism and a deep bite are treated by means of mandibular advancement, there is in some cases a discongruity between the incisal pathway and the condylar path along the articular eminence. Signs and symptoms of 'closed-lock' may then occur (figure 3). When patients with relative mandibular retrognathism are treated by means of superior repositioning of the maxilla, the angle of the condyle relative to the articular eminence becomes steep due to autorotation (figure 4).[8-11] In cases of absolute mandibular retrognathism with high mandibular plane angle where a bimaxillary procedure is indicated for reasons of stability, it is not always possible to maintain the condylar fragment in its original position. Some autorotation must occur to prevent the need for an osteosynthesis between the upper border of the

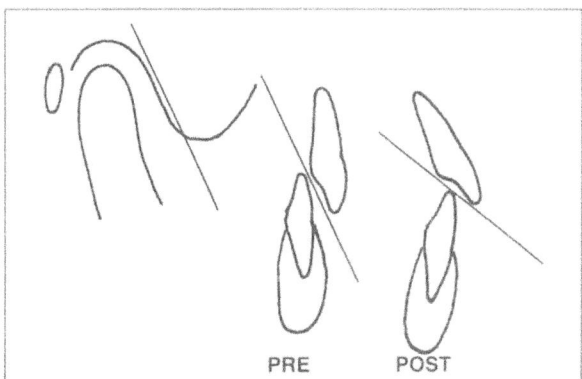

Figure 3.
Discongruency between steepness of articular eminence and incisal pathway after surgical correction of the deep bite in cases of mandibular retrognathism with closed bite.

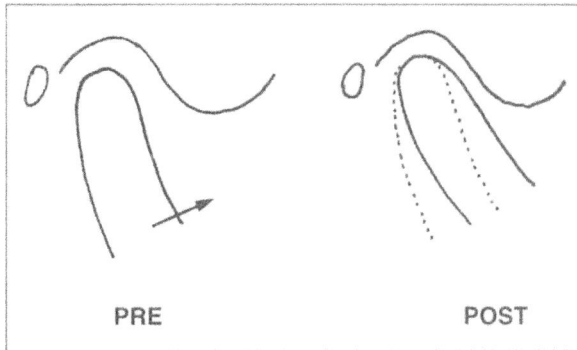

Figure 4.
As a result of autorotation of the mandible, the glenoid fossa becomes relatively deeper and the articular eminence relatively steeper.

condylar fragment and the lower border of the mandibular body (figure 5). This has the same effect of steepening the angle of the condyle relative to the articular eminence as previously mentioned.

Occasionally, the anatomical configuration of the condyle gives rise to more than one rotation point, which may complicate the positioning of the maxilla in the correction of relative mandibular retrognathism. In the first traject of rotation, the most posterior condylar area serves as rotation center, while in a more closed position the anterior edge distracts the first rotation center out of the fossa (figure 6).

In instances of hypermobility of the temporomandibular joint disc it is possible that the disc may become displaced anterior to the condylar head following an orthognathic procedure using intermaxillary fixation. Following release of the intermaxillary fixation, the displaced disc may cause restricted mouth opening.

The volume and anatomical configuration of the condylar head differ from one deformity to another. In cases with a low mandibular plane angle, condylar growth is considered to be directed more anteriorly than in cases with a high mandibular plane angle. This appears to influence the behaviour of the joint following orthognathic surgery.[12,13]

Figure 5.
In bimaxillary surgery it is
not always possible to maintain the condylar fragment
in the original position.
Some autorotation must occur to prevent the need for
an osteosynthesis between
the upper border of the condylar fragment and the
lower border of the mandibular body.

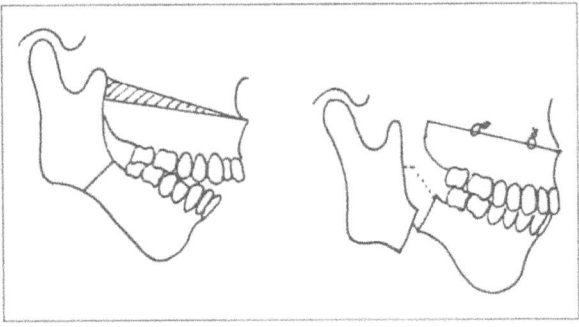

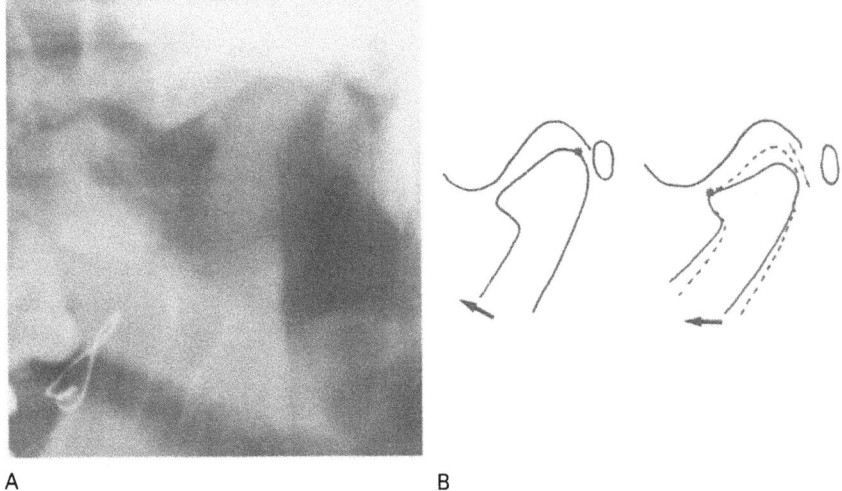

A   B

Figure 6.
Two rotation points related to condylar configuration.
A. Radiograph of condyle.
B. In the first traject of autorotation the most posterior area serves as rotation center. In a more closed
position the anterior edge distracts this area out of the fossa.

Finally, forced opening of the mouth during either intubation or the surgical
procedure can in itself produce joint problems.

Behaviour of the temporomandibular joint related to orthognathic surgery

Kerstens et al. studied the temporomandibular joints of patients who underwent
orthognathic surgery in the period from 1982 to 1987.[2] The data obtained appear
to be consistent over the last seven years. Of the 480 patients who underwent
orthognathic surgery, 16% (78 patients) reported pre-operative signs and symp-

toms of temporomandibular disorders. As studies of a 'normal' population show an incidence of temporomandibular joint dysfunction between 14% and 16%, the orthognathic group under study had a 'normal' incidence of temporo-mandibular joint dysfunction.[14-16] Following orthognathic surgery, 66% of the individuals with pre-existing temporomandibular joint problems reported im-provement of their symptoms (52 patients). However, 14% of the patients who had no problems pre-operatively developed temporomandibular joint pain and dysfunction following orthognathic surgery. When considering the total group, no real changes occurred. However, when the results are analyzed for each of the five deformity types, more information is obtained about the behaviour of the temporomandibular joint.

Mandibular prognathism without open bite (75 patients)
Pre-operatively, 12% (9 patients) had temporomandibular joint pain and dys-function. Post-operatively, the number of patients who continued to have problems dropped to 9% (7 patients), indicating a slight improvement. These findings are more or less in accordance with data in the literature.[17,18]

Mandibular prognathism with open bite (77 patients)
Pre-operatively, 12% (9 patients) showed temporomandibular joint signs and symptoms, and post-operatively this increased to 16%, which is within 'normal' limits.

Mandibular retrognathism with low/normal mandibular plane angle
(162 patients)
Pre-operatively, 22% (35 patients) showed temporomandibular joint dysfunc-tion, representing a higher than normal prevalence. Post-operatively, 7% (12 patients) continued to complain of temporomandibular joint symptoms, indi-cating a considerable decrease, which supports previous findings in the litera-ture.[19,20]

Relative mandibular retrognathism with high mandibular plane angle
(85 patients)
Pre-operatively, 13 patients (15%) showed temporomandibular joint symp-toms, and this percentage remained unchanged post-operatively. In the litera-ture there is no consistency regarding this group.[8-10]

Absolute mandibular retrognathism with high mandibular plane angle
(81 patients)
Pre-operatively, 15% (12 patients) had signs and symptoms of temporo-mandibular disorders. Post-operatively, 5 patients reported that the symptoms had remained unchanged or had increased. Fourteen patients who had no pre-operative symptoms developed temporomandibular joint pain and dysfunc-tion post-operatively. Thus, 19 patients (23%) complained of temporomandibu-lar joint dysfunction. In this group, radiographic evidence of condylar resorp-

Figure 7.
Condylar resorption after surgical orthodontic correction of absolute mandibular retrognathism.

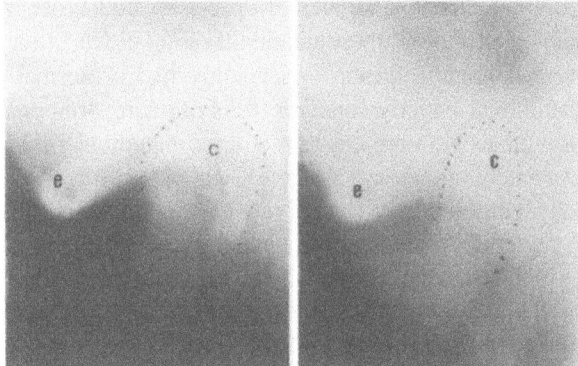

tion is sometimes seen (figure 7). The etiology of this phenomenon is unclear.[21-23] Research concerning the influence of intermaxillary immobilization on the joint and the value of the pre-operative radiographic examination is currently being carried out.[24,25]

We can conclude from these results that in patients with a low/normal mandibular plane angle orthognathic surgery may result in an improvement of the existing temporomandibular joint dysfunction (66%). The use of internal fixation in order to avoid intermaxillary fixation appears to a large extent to prevent the occurrence of an internal derangement with a permanent disc displacement. In cases of absolute mandibular retrognathism with high mandibular plane angle there is a chance that the complaints of temporomandibular joint dysfunction will increase and that condylar resorption, leading to relapse, will occur. Although the use of internal fixation instead of intermaxillary fixation significantly reduces the occurrence of condylar resorption, this adverse phenomenon still occurs (in 11% of the cases) and must be discussed with the patient beforehand.

Temporomandibular joint and osteotomy recommendations

The following protocol is recommended in patients with temporomandibular joint disorders in combination with a dentofacial deformity. When the complaints resolve after appropriate non-surgical treatment, surgical orthodontic correction may be considered in all deformity categories. In cases of absolute mandibular retrognathism with high mandibular plane angle, the benefit of orthognathic surgery must be carefully weighed against the potential adverse effects on the temporomandibular joint. Pre-operative psychological evaluation is strongly advised.

Relative anatomical discrepancies, e.g., resulting from autorotation or discongruity of the steepness of the articular eminence and the incisal pathway, may necessitate continuation of occlusal appliance therapy post-operatively. In addition, physical therapy can be very beneficial in rehabilitating the joint.[26,27] If complaints remain despite these precautions, temporomandibular arthroscopy or even surgery may be indicated.[28] Simultaneous joint surgery and orthognathic surgery is not advised.

References

1 Tuinzing DB, Greebe RB, Dorenbos J, Van der Kwast WAM. Surgical Orthodontics. Diagnosis and Treatment. Amsterdam: Free University Press, 1993
2 Kerstens HCJ, Tuinzing DB, Van der Kwast WAM. Temporomandibular joint symptoms in orthognathic surgery. J Cranio Max Fac Surg 1989; 17:215
3 Greebe RB. Stabiliteit en recidief na chirurgische verplaatsing van de onderkaak. Thesis, Free University of Amsterdam, The Netherlands, 1987
4 Hakman CJ. Een nieuw gezicht? Thesis, Free University of Amsterdam, The Netherlands, 1993
5 Storum KA, Bell WH. Hypomobility after maxillary and mandibular osteotomies. Oral Surg Oral Med Oral Pathol 1984; 57:7
6 Friedman MH, Weisberg J, Weber FL. Postsurgical temporomandibular joint hypomobility; rehabilitation technique. Oral Surg Oral Med Oral Path 1993; 75:24
7 Kerstens HCJ, Tuinzing DB, Golding RP, Van der Kwast WAM. The inclination of the temporomandibular joint eminence and internal derangement. Int J Oral Maxillofac Surg 1989; 18:229
8 Herbosa EG, Rotskoff KS, Ramos BF, Ambrookian HS. Condylar position in superior maxillary repositioning and its effects on the temporomandibular joint. J Oral Maxillofac Surg 1990; 48:690
9 Kahnberg KE. TMJ complications associated with superior repositioning of the maxilla. J Craniomandibular Pract 1988; 6:312
10 de Mol van Otterloo JJ, Dorenbos J, Tuinzing DB, van der Kwast WAM. TMJ performance and behaviour in patients more than 6 years after le Fort I osteotomy. Br J Oral Maxillofac Surg 1993; 31:83
11 O'Ryan F, Epker BN. Surgical orthodontics and the temporomandibular joint. I. Superior repositioning of the maxilla. Am J Orthod 1983; 83:408
12 O'Ryan F, Epker BN. Temporomandibular joint function and morphology: observation on the spectra of normalcy. Oral Surg Oral Med Oral Pathol 1984; 58:272
13 Dibbets JMH. Juvenile temporomandibular joint dysfunction and craniofacial growth. Thesis, University of Groningen, The Netherlands, 1977
14 Laskin DM, Ryan WA, Greene CS. Incidence of temporomandibular symptoms in patients with major skeletal malocclusions: a survey of oral and maxillofacial surgery training programs. Oral Surg Oral Med Oral Pathol 1986; 61:537
15 Solberg WK, Woo MW, Houston JB. Prevalence of mandibular dysfunction in young adults. J Am Dent Assoc 1979; 98:25
16 Link JJ, Nickerson Jr. JW. Temporomandibular joint internal derangements in an orthognathic surgery population. Int J Adult Orthod Orthognath Surg 1992; 7:161
17 Nagamine T, Kobayashi T, Nakajima T, Hanada K. The effects of surgical-orthodontic correction of skeletal class III malocclusion on mandibular movement. J Oral Maxillofac Surg 1993; 51:385
18 Wisth PJ. Mandibular function and dysfunction in patients with mandibular prognathism. Am J Orthod 1984; 85:193
19 Piecuch J, Tideman H, de Koomen HA. Short-face syndrome: treatment of myofacial pain dysfunction by maxillary dysimpaction. Oral Surg Oral Med Oral Pathol 1980; 49:112
20 Van Sickels JE, Ivey DW. Myofacial pain dysfunction: a manifestation of the short-face syndrome. J Prosthet Dent 1979; 42:547
21 Chuong R, Piper MA. Avascular necrosis of the mandibular condyle. Pathogenesis and concepts of management. Oral Surg Oral Med Oral Path 1993; 75:428
22 Kerstens HCJ, Tuinzing DB, Golding RP, Van der Kwast WAM. Condylar atrophy and osteoarthrosis after bimaxillary surgery. Oral Surg Oral Med Oral Pathol 1990; 67:274
23 Moore KE, Gooris PJJ, Stoelinga PJW. The contributing role of condylar resorption to skeletal relapse following mandibular advancement surgery: report of five cases. J Oral Maxillofac Surg 1991; 49:448

24 Schellhas KP, Wilkes CH, Fritts HM, et al. Temporomandibular joint: MR imaging of internal derangements and postoperative changes. AJNR 1987; 8:1093
25 Bouwman JPB, Tuinzing DB, Kerstens HCJ. Condylar resorption in orthognathic surgery. The role of intermaxillary fixation. Oral Surg Oral Med Oral Pathol 1994; 78:138
26 Bell WH, Gonyea W, Finn RA, et al. Muscular rehabilitation after orthognathic surgery. Oral Surg Oral Med Oral Pathol 1983; 56:229
27 Lafferty Braun B. The effect of physical therapy intervention on incisal opening after temporo-mandibular joint surgery. Oral Surg Oral Med Oral Path 1987; 64:544
28 Stegenga B, de Bont LGM, Dijkstra PU, Boering G. Short-term outcome of arthroscopic surgery of the temporomandibular joint osteoarthrosis and internal derangement. Br J Oral Maxillofac Surg 1993; 31:3

Management of Temporomandibular
Joint Degenerative Diseases
ed. by B. Stegenga & L.G.M. de Bont
© 1996 Birkhäuser Verlag Basel/Switzerland

Criteria for temporomandibular joint treatment outcome

Anders B. Holmlund

*Department of Oral and Maxillofacial Surgery, School of Dentistry, Karolinska Institutet,
14104 Huddinge, Sweden*

Summary: Most follow-up studies of surgical and non-surgical treatment of temporomandibular joint
degenerative diseases are retrospective and do not specify inclusion and exclusion criteria, methods of
assessment, outcome criteria, or the number of patients drop-outs. Recommendations with regard to
study design are given, with special reference to temporomandibular joint degenerative diseases.

Introduction

Medical history shows several examples of how highly regarded surgical or
non-surgical methods based on empiricism are later relegated in well-designed
controlled studies to methods of historical significance only. Methods for the
treatment of temporomandibular disorders are no exception. The reasons for
this are many. Most common is the confusion regarding the diagnosis of
temporomandibular disorders, which has existed for a long time and is reflected
in the literature by expressions like 'pain-dysfunction syndrome' or 'craniomandibular dysfunction'. In most studies, the difficulty of making a specific
diagnosis and the resulting inability to include the right patients have produced
results that cannot be compared with those of other studies. Recently, this
problem has been addressed extensively.[1,2] A classification of temporomandibular disorders has been proposed which agrees with that used for other
musculoskeletal disorders.[1] Other difficulties have included inadequate design
and inadequate follow-up studies.[1,3,4] It is the aim of this chapter to review the
available literature and provide suggestions for improving the evaluation of
treatment outcome.

Requirements for treatment outcome evaluation

A properly conducted follow-up study should specify the aims of treatment, be
prospective, specify inclusion and exclusion criteria, use proper methods of
assessment, and have well-defined criteria for outcome evaluation, an adequate
follow-up period, a minimal number of drop-outs, and appropriate statistical
analysis.

Biological and clinical objectives of treatment

The optimal goals of surgical and non-surgical treatment include elimination of disease or deformity, restoration of anatomy and function, and relief of symptoms. When evaluating the aims in treating patients with temporo-mandibular joint degenerative diseases, one should consider the disease process and the sequence of the various procedures. Temporomandibular joint degenerative diseases are rarely associated with major deformities, and usually the prognosis for spontaneous long-term remission is good.[5] However, during the course of the disease episodes of pain and impaired mandibular function often occur. Furthermore, it seems impossible to predict the length of this symptomatic period in the individual patient, and thus treatment is often needed. Since the etiology and pathogenesis are not yet fully understood, the least treatment that benefits the patient should be provided. Information and reassurance of the patient are always important, as is the patient's consent to the proposed treatment. As a rule, non-surgical treatment should precede surgery but should not be unnecessarily prolonged if unsuccessful.

Since causal therapy is not feasible, more specific aims in treating temporo-mandibular joint degenerative diseases include biological aims, i.e., to arrest the disease and to promote residual healing and adaptation capacity, and clinical aims, i.e., to gain the patient's cooperation, to alleviate pain, and to improve mandibular function.

Study design

The treatment can be evaluated with or without the use of scientific methods. When we rely on our clinical experience, inherent weaknesses become evident. First, the experience of many clinicians varies greatly, and, second, there is always a risk of subjective upgrading of the post-operative recordings.[6] Most clinicians of course know this and instead rely on follow-up studies. Unfortunately, the methods used in such studies are also frequently subjective and empirical. The literature shows many examples of follow-up studies that do not specify inclusion and exclusion criteria, methods of assessment, and outcome criteria. The recent failures of some temporomandibular joint implants are warning examples. Retrospective studies have definite limitations. Frequently, more than one surgeon has been involved, and the drop-out frequency in many studies is unacceptably high. A prospective study design is, therefore, preferable.

Evaluation of patient treatment outcome is best performed in randomized clinical trials.[7] Random allocation of patients reduces the risk of selection bias inherent to uncontrolled or non-randomized studies, and provides more reliable data with regard to differences in outcome. Randomized studies usually require approval by a research ethics committee, and more formal consent by the patient. Problems may therefore arise. First, if considerable differences exist between the methods to be compared, e.g., comparison of a surgical and a non-surgical treatment, the patient may fail to understand why the medical experts are so uncertain about how to treat the disease. Second, in life-threatening diseases, e.g., malignant tumors, the choice of treatment may place an additional burden on the participants. This, of course, is not applicable to temporomandibular disorders. A much more common problem is that clinicians have a preference for one of the treatment alternatives. Thus they may be willing to take part in a randomized trial only if they are totally uncertain about the new treatment. However, the history of medicine shows several examples of treatments previously regarded as efficient which later, in randomized clinical trials, have proved ineffective. The problem of clinicians' preference can be solved either by making them less certain (providing them with information on research that argues against the preferred method) or by random assignment to more than one clinician. If a widely used and accepted surgical or non-surgical method exists, then the new procedure should be compared with this method.

Another problem in many studies is that the treatment frequently is not a single procedure but a combination of different procedures. For example, in many studies involving arthroscopic surgery, the surgical procedure is combined with intra-articular injections of steroids and immediately followed by physical therapy. An optimal design avoids additional treatments, as far as this is ethically possible.

Inclusion and exclusion criteria

Inclusion criteria
The inclusion of patients in a treatment outcome study should be based on defined diagnostic criteria. Unfortunately, the clinical signs and symptoms of many temporomandibular disorders frequently overlap. Crepitus correlates with arthroscopic features of advanced osteoarthrosis.[8] However, no such correlation was found for joints with early-phase osteoarthrosis.[8] Locking is frequently associated with temporomandibular joint osteoarthrosis,[9] but it may also be found in joints without degenerative changes.[10,11] Reciprocal clicking seems to correlate with little, if any, osteoarthrosis.[8] Radiographic features, such as flattening, sclerosis, osteophytes, and erosions have been thought to reflect degenerative changes in the temporomandibular joint.[12] Erosions seem to be the most reliable radiographic feature.[13,14] However, no distinction can be made between active and "burned-out" osteoarthrosis on the basis of these features. Furthermore, a correlation with clinical signs depends on the degree of condylar translation.[13] The grading system for evaluation of radiographs, as advocated by Rohlin,[15] seems most appropriate. Corrected sagittal and frontal tomography is better than plain radiography,[16] arthrography, and magnetic resonance imaging.[17] Arthroscopy offers unique diagnostic information and shows high accuracy with osteoarthrosis and inflammation.[9,11,18] Arthroscopic criteria for osteoarthrosis and inflammation have been proposed,[9,11,18] and

biopsies of cartilage and synovium can readily be taken. A disadvantage is that the lower compartment is difficult to explore. Except for interference from remodeling mainly located on the condyle,[19] pathologic activity in the lower compartment is usually reflected in the upper compartment. Arthroscopy is also uniquely useful for assessing the various stages of the disease process, and it is therefore probably the ideal method for determining the inclusion of patients with temporomandibular joint degenerative diseases. For obvious reasons this approach is not applicable to non-surgical treatment, but it should be considered when surgery is involved.

Evaluating treatments for temporomandibular disorders is a complex subject, but the complexity becomes even greater if we fail to use proper inclusion criteria. The need for regular international consensus meetings must be emphasized.[20]

If treatment involves surgery, proper non-surgical treatment should always precede surgery and should be the first inclusion criterion. It is also essential to ensure that the pain comes from the diseased temporomandibular joint, especially if surgery is planned. Therefore, a second inclusion criterion may be that diagnostic local anesthesia should definitely alleviate arthralgia.

Exclusion criteria

Also important are the exclusion criteria, which may include diseases and malformations that can affect the temporomandibular joint or surrounding tissues. Among these are chronic arthritis, regional non-articular disorders, and growth disturbances. Another category consists of psychological disorders involving chronic pain. Patients with such problems may be detected with appropriate measures.[1] A third category may comprise patients with an inability to keep follow-up appointments. Other relative criteria for exclusion may concern patients with an extremely long duration of symptoms, previous treatments, and parafunctional habits. Most important, however, is a specification of the exclusion criteria used.

Methods of assessment

The most common complaints of patients with temporomandibular disorders are joint and muscle pain during mandibular movements, impaired mandibular function, and, to a much lesser extent, disturbing joint sounds.

To evaluate anamnestic pain, basic information concerning pain complaints (e.g., Global Pain Impact scale[1]) and the effect of pain on daily functioning and general well-being can be assessed. Helkimo's dysfunction index[21] has been used in several follow-up studies. This index was designed originally for epidemiological studies and is not relevant to treatment outcome evaluation. Another general index (the craniomandibular index) was developed by Fricton and Schiffman.[22] Recently, an index with good clinimetric properties has been developed to evaluate functional impairment of mandibular function (Mandibular Function Impairment Questionnaire).[1] It seems to be a simple and reliable instrument for assessing the degree of functional impairment without measuring clinical signs and symptoms in patients with temporomandibular joint osteoarthrosis and internal derangement.

Pain assessment always involves subjective features. The use of a visual analog scale can make the evaluation of pain less subjective. The baseline intensity level of pain at rest is recorded and compared with changes in pain level in response to the various mandibular movements. Pre-operative and post-operative recordings are then compared.

Signs and symptoms such as joint and muscle tenderness and joint sounds are not very reliable. Many clinicians also know that these clinical signs and symptoms may change spontaneously over time. Clinical assessment of joint and muscle tenderness is best performed with digital palpation. Devices for more standardized "palpation" (so-called algometers) may improve reliability.[23] Assessment of pain in response to muscle palpation is only moderately reliable.[24] Furthermore, intra-observer variation in such recordings is lower than the variation between observers.[24,25] The clinical examination should therefore be performed by a single, well-trained clinician. If several clinicians are involved, calibration of the examiners is important. For practical reasons, the clinician often evaluates the outcome of treatment himself. In this setting, the clinical assessment may be biased by an unknown upgrading of the post-operative recordings.[6] Therefore, evaluation of treatment outcome by a fellow clinician may be a better alternative.

Temporomandibular joint sounds may be investigated clinically by means of digital palpation or a stethoscope. However, both methods seem to have only marginal reliability.[24] Joints sounds are best detected on vertical opening.[24]

The assessment of mandibular mobility includes measurement of vertical and horizontal movements. However, linear mouth opening, i.e., the maximum interincisal distance added to the vertical overlap of the dentition, shows only a weak correlation with condylar mobility as measured on transpharyngeal radiograms.[2] A more accurate procedure, which also is independent of mandibular length, is to measure the angle of mouth opening.[2] However, measuring linear mouth opening is simple and very reliable,[2,24] and is therefore an excellent method for clinical follow-up studies. Angular mouth opening is the method of choice for epidemiological research or when temporomandibular joint mobility is compared with the mobility of other joints.[2] The assessment of horizontal, i.e., protrusive and laterotrusive mandibular, movements is less reliable.[24] Clinically, the sliding capacity of the joint may best be assessed during protrusion and subsequent maximum opening.[1] Deviation of the mandible on maximum opening may indicate restricted joint translation, but may be difficult to distinguish from extra-articular causes such as enlargement of the coronoid process or fibrosis of the muscle tendons.

Several instruments for clinical assessment have been proposed, including electromyography, sonography, Doppler auscultation, and jaw-tracing devices. These devices seem to have limited clinical value or to yield insufficient scientific data.

Among the radiographic techniques, corrected tomography (and computerized tomography) seem to provide the most accurate diagnostic information. An acceptable reproducibility has been achieved with most radiographic techniques, provided that a cephalostat is used.[16] Radiographic examination does not necessarily provide information on disease activity. However, the degree of condylar mobility is readily assessed on tomograms and possibly also on transpharyngeal and transcranial projections. As with clinical assessment, intra-observer variation is lower than variation between observers, and radiographic interpretations should therefore be made by a single well-trained radiologist.[26] If more observers participate, a long calibration period is recommended.[27]

Arthrography and magnetic resonance imaging may be useful for demonstrating soft tissue changes in the temporomandibular joint, e.g., successful or unsuccessful repositioning of the temporomandibular joint disc following arthrotomy or arthroscopic surgery. Neither soft tissue nor hard tissue imaging necessarily correlates with pain or even with impaired mandibular function.[28]

Arthroscopy is potentially of great value in the evaluation of disease activity. It is the author's firm conviction that no other method opens up such possibilities. Furthermore, simultaneous biopsy permits correlation between visual observations and the changes occurring in the tissues. As previously mentioned, the diagnostic accuracy of temporomandibular joint arthroscopy is high in osteoarthrosis and inflammation.[9,11,18] Future aims must be to reinforce arthroscopic diagnostic criteria by correlating them to molecular markers for disease activity.

From a clinical point of view, joint tenderness and pain on mandibular movements have shown a weak but significant correlation with arthroscopic synovitis.[8,29] As previously mentioned, pain may change spontaneously during the course of treatment. Mechanisms other than classic inflammation, such as the release of neuropeptides, may also be important.[10] More systematic arthroscopic investigations are highly recommended.

Outcome criteria

The American Association of Oral and Maxillofacial Surgeons has proposed the following criteria for successful treatment:[30]

- pain absent or so mild, brief, and infrequent as to be of no concern to the patient
- range of motion greater than 35 mm for vertical and greater than 6 mm for protrusive and lateral excursions
- regular diet which, at worst, avoids tough or hard foods – patient minimally inconvenienced by diet
- radiographic changes in joint unimportant unless there are severe destructive changes
- absence of significant complications.

However, there are weaknesses associated with these criteria. For instance, measurements of 35 mm for vertical and 6 mm for horizontal mandibular movements do not emanate from findings in epidemiologic studies. In some patients with temporomandibular joint degenerative diseases (e.g., internal derangement with periodic locking), the vertical and horizontal movements exceed 35 mm and 6 mm, respectively. Post-operative values may therefore be lower than pre-operative values and still represent a successful case according to the above-mentioned criteria. These criteria have frequently been used in follow-up studies and seem to correlate with the patient's feeling of well-being and good mandibular function,[19,31] and a consensus exists for their use in outcome evaluation in individual patients and in more ordinary follow-up studies.[20] In research, the previously mentioned methods for anamnestic and clinical assessment of pain and functional impairment should be employed instead. The recommendations for the various cut-off points for pain and functional impairment, recently described by Stegenga,[1,32] seem very appropriate.

Complications may occur with any treatment, but they seem to be mainly associated with surgery. Such complications may be intra-operative (e.g., persistent bleeding or iatrogenic damage) or post-operative (e.g., nerve damage, infection, deafness, unesthetic scar). Complication rates for arthroscopic surgery and discectomy without implants have been low.[19,31] If reconstructive surgery and implants are involved, much higher complication rates must be expected. If permanent unfavorable sequelae remain, the case must be regarded as a treatment failure. Informed patient consent to all treatments, especially surgery, is mandatory.

End-points, drop-outs, and statistical analysis

It is questionable whether criteria for a favorable outcome should require long-lasting functional improvement and pain relief. Regarding arthritides this may not be possible, since the etiology and pathogenesis are not well understood. For example, in knee joints affected by rheumatoid arthritis, arthroscopic synovectomy may bring an improvement for a few years, but then the symptoms recur.[33] On the other hand, the treatment can induce changes that camouflage the symptoms. In temporomandibular joint open surgery denervation always occurs to some extent. During the period of nerve regeneration, symptoms may be absent but may recur after nerve regeneration is completed, usually within a year.

Only a few studies have tried to analyze the characteristics of an unsuccessful result. One problem in most temporomandibular joint follow-up studies is that the frequencies of unsuccessful results in patients are so low that it is almost impossible to perform a thorough investigation of possible negative factors. A few prospective temporomandibular joint discectomy studies in patients with or without macroscopic degenerative disease, however, indicate that failures develop early in the follow-up period (usually within the first six months), and that patients considered to have improved considerably on a short-term basis continue to do so in the long term.[19,31] On the other hand, studies involving disc-substituting implants indicate the need for a longer follow-up.[34]

Too many follow-up studies on temporomandibular disorders give no information about drop-out frequencies. Patients are more or less stable as regards their way of life. In the United States where people move around considerably, it is not unusual for patients to seek medical treatment far from their place of residence. In Europe, people are more stable in this respect, and patients in a follow-up study therefore can easily be asked to return for another examination. Many patients in the United States go to another clinician if the first treatment proves unsatisfactory, while European patients more often continue to go to the same clinician. A large number of drop-outs reduces the validity of the follow-up study. The drop-out frequency must be reported in a follow-up study and be statistically evaluated.

Finally, an appropriate statistical analysis is the only good source of information as to whether the influence of chance has been underestimated.

Recommendations

Clinical evaluation

For clinical follow-up the following recommendations are proposed:

– prospective pre- and post-operative recordings
– standardized techniques for clinical examination (joint auscultation, joint and muscle palpation, measurements of vertical and horizontal mandibular movements)
– outcome criteria according to the American Association of Oral and Maxillofacial Surgeons.

Clinical research

Based on the information provided in this chapter, the following are recommended for formal clinical research:

– randomized clinical trials
– specific inclusion and exclusion criteria
– valid and reliable assessment of pain and mandibular function, standardized techniques for clinical examination, assessment of hard and soft tissue pathology (plain film, computerized tomography, magnetic resonance imaging, and arthroscopy)
– follow-up period for arthroscopic surgery, disc repositioning, and discec-

tomy without alloplastic implants of at least one year; unlimited follow-up for discectomy with alloplastic implants (provided the biocompatibility of the implant has been thoroughly tested) and for arthroplasty.

References

1 Stegenga B. Temporomandibular joint osteoarthrosis and internal derangement. Diagnostic and therapeutic outcome assessment. Thesis, University of Groningen, The Netherlands, 1991
2 Dijkstra PU. Temporomandibular joint: Osteoarthrosis and joint mobility. Thesis, University of Groningen, The Netherlands, 1993
3 Smith JP. Methodology in a sample of the temporomandibular joint literature. J Dent 1986; 14:70
4 Holmlund A. Surgery for TMJ internal derangement. Evaluation of treatment outcome and criteria for success. Int J Oral Maxillofac Surg 1993; 22:75
5 Rasmussen OC. Temporomandibular arthropathy. Clinical, radiologic, and therapeutic aspects, with emphasis on diagnosis. Int J Oral Surg 1983; 12:365
6 Wulff HR. Rationel klinik. 2nd ed. Copenhagen: Munksgaard, 1981; 153
7 Korn EL, Baumrind S. Randomized clinical trials with clinician preferred treatment. Lancet 1992; 337:149
8 Holmlund A, Hellsing G, Axelsson S. The temporomandibular joint: A comparison of clinical and arthroscopic findings. J Prosthet Dent 1989; 62:61
9 Holmlund A, Gynther GW, Reinholt FP. Disk derangement and inflammatory changes in the posterior disk attachment of the temporomandibular joint. A histologic study. Oral Surg Oral Med Oral Pathol 1992; 73:9
10 Holmlund A, Ekblom A, Hansson P, Lind J, Lundeberg T, Theodorsson E. Concentrations of neuropeptides substance P, neurokinin A, calcitonin gene-related peptide, neuropeptide Y and vasoactive intestinal polypeptide in synovial fluid of the human temporomandibular joint. A correlation with symptoms, signs and arthroscopic findings. Int J Oral Maxillofac Surg 1991; 20:228
11 Holmlund A, Gynther G, Reinholt FP. Rheumatoid arthritis and disk derangement of the temporomandibular joint. A comparative arthroscopic study. Oral Surg Oral Med Oral Pathol 1992; 73:273
12 Rohlin M, Akerman S, Kopp S. Tomography as an aid to detect macroscopic changes of the temporomandibular joint: an autopsy study of the aged. Acta Odontol Scand 1986; 44:131
13 Akerman S, Kopp S. Nilner M, Peterson A, Rohlin M. Relationship between clinical and radiologic findings of the temporomandibular joint in rheumatoid arthritis..Oral Surg Oral Med Oral Pathol 1988; 66:639
14 Goupille P, Fouquet B, Cotty P, Goga D, Mateu J, Valat J-P. The temporomandibular joint in rheumatoid arthritis. Correlations between clinical and computed tomography features. J Rheumatol 1990; 17:1285
15 Rohlin M, Petersson A. Rheumatoid arthritis of the temporomandibular joint: Radiologic evaluation based on standard references films. Oral Surg Oral Med Oral Pathol 1989; 67:594
16 Petersson A. Radiography of the temporomandibular joint. A comparison of information obtained from different radiographic techniques. Thesis, University of Malmö, Sweden, 1976
17 Watt-Smith S, Sadler A, Baddeley H, Renton P. Comparison of arthrotomographic and magnetic resonance imaging of 50 temporomandibular joints with operative findings. Br J Oral Maxillofac Surg 1993; 31:139
18 Holmlund A. Diagnostic accuracy of temporomandibular joint arthroscopy. A comparison of findings during arthroscopy and arthrotomy. Oral Maxillofac Surg Clin North Am 1989; 1:79
19 Holmlund A, Gynther G, Axelsson S. Diskectomy in treatment of internal derangement of the temporomandibular joint. Follow-up at 1, 3, and 5 years. Oral Surg Oral Med Oral Pathol 1993; 76:266
20 Goss AN. Towards an international consensus on temporomandibular joint surgery. Report of the Second International Consensus Meeting, April 1992, Buenos Aires, Argentina. Int J Oral Maxillofac Surg 1993; 22:78
21 Helkimo M. Studies on function and dysfunction of the masticatory system. III. Analysis of anamnestic and clinical recordings of dysfunction with the aid of indices. Swed Dent J 1974; 67:165
22 Fricton JR, Schiffman EL. The craniomandibular index: validity. J Prosthet Dent 1987; 58:222

23 Chung S-C, Um B-Y, Kim H-S. Evaluation of pressure pain threshold in head and neck muscles by electronic algometer: intrarater and interrater reliability. J Craniomandibular Pract 1992; 10:28

24 Dworkin SF, LeResche L, DeRouen T, Von Korff M. Assessing clinical signs of temporomandibular disorders: reliability of clinical examiners. J Prosthet Dent 1990; 63:574

25 Carlsson GE, Egermarkt-Eriksson I, Magnusson T. Intra- and interobserver variation in functional examination of the masticatory system. Swed Dent J 1980; 4:187

26 Kopp S, Rockler B. Variation in interpretation of radiographs of temporomandibular and hand joints. Dentomaxillofac Radiol 1978; 7:95

27 Tasaki M, Westesson P-L. Observer performance in interpretation of MR images of the temporomandibular joint. Oral Surg Oral Med Oral Pathol 1993; 75:528

28 Montgomery MT, Van Sickels JE, Harms SE. Success of temporomandibular joint arthroscopy in disk displacement with and without reduction. Oral Surg Oral Med Oral Pathol 1991; 71:651

29 Murakami K-I, Segami N, Fujimura K, Iizuka T. Correlation between pain and synovitis in patients with internal derangement of the temporomandibular joint. J Oral Maxillofac Surg 1991; 49:1159

30 Dolwick MF. 1984 criteria for TMJ meniscus surgery. Chicago: Am Assoc Oral Maxillofac Surg, 1984

31 Eriksson L, Westesson P-L. Temporomandibular joint diskectomy. No positive effect of temporary silicone implants in a 5-year follow-up. Oral Surg Oral Med Oral Pathol 1992; 74:259

32 Stegenga B, de Bont LGM, Dijkstra PU, Boering G. Short-term outcome of arthroscopic surgery of the temporomandibular joint osteoarthrosis and internal derangement: a randomized controlled clinical trial. Br J Oral Maxillofac Surg 1993; 31:3

33 Goldie I. A synopsis of surgery for rheumatoid arthritis (excluding the hand). Clin Orthop 1984; 191:185

34 Feinerman DM, Piecuch JF. Long-term retrospective analysis of twenty-three Proplast-Teflon temporomandibular joint interpositional implants. Int J Oral Maxillofac Surg 1993; 22:11

Management of Temporomandibular
Joint Degenerative Diseases
ed. by B. Stegenga & L.G.M. de Bont
© 1996 Birkhäuser Verlag Basel/Switzerland

The current role of conventional radiography and computerized tomography in temporomandibular joint treatment planning

Bart van der Kuijl

*Department of Oral and Maxillofacial Surgery, University Hospital Groningen, 9700 RB Groningen,
The Netherlands*

Summary: Conventional radiography still has a place in the diagnosis and treatment planning of
temporomandibular disorders. Direct sagittal computerized tomography is very effective in determining
changes of condylar shape and position, and of the articular eminence. It appears to be the proper imaging
modality in differential diagnostic cases in which a more extended and complex disorder is suggested
but not clearly documented on conventional radiographs.

Introduction

Diagnostic imaging is important for establishing a correct diagnosis, for documentation, and for treatment evaluation of temporomandibular disorders.[1,2] A wide range of imaging techniques is available, including conventional ('plain film') radiography, tomography, arthrography, fluoroscopy, computerized tomography, magnetic resonance imaging, and radionuclide imaging.[3]

Conventional radiography

Conventional radiography still has its place in the diagnostic process, and cannot simply be omitted because of the availability of, usually far more expensive, modern techniques. At our department, the panoramic technique, the transcranial lateral oblique technique according to Schüller, the transpharyngeal infracranial technique according to Parma, and cephalometric techniques have been used for more than 30 years for routine examination of the temporomandibular joint.[4] Although improvements have been made, including faster films, more powerful intensifier screens, and state-of-the-art X-ray machines, the original projection parameters of the Schüller and Parma techniques remained the same, enabling reliable follow-up of degenerative processes in single patients as well as long-term research on the natural course and treatment outcome of osteoarthrosis of the temporomandibular joint.[5]

Panoramic X-ray

The panoramic X-ray (figure 1) is primarily used for screening oral and maxillofacial disorders. The technique is valuable in the differential diagnosis of complex pain problems. Odontogenic and other non-articular causes of craniofacial pain can be excluded before specific diagnostic procedures for temporomandibular disorders are initiated. It offers a great amount of diagnostic information in a single, easy and fast to produce film, representing upper and lower jaws, temporomandibular joints, maxillary sinuses, and the dentition. The image of the temporomandibular joints, however, is not as reliable and reproducible as with transcranial and transpharyngeal techniques.

Figure 1.
Panoramic radiograph.

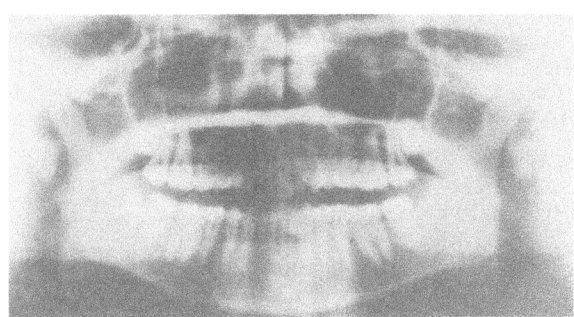

Transcranial X-ray

The transcranial X-ray (according to Schüller, figure 2) is made using a highly reproducible technique on an isocentric medical X-ray machine, especially designed for skull radiography. The patient is sitting in an adjusted dental chair, mounted to a crossed-rail construction for precise alignment of the joint in the isocenter of the apparatus. The projection is made with the dentition in habitual occlusion. The X-ray beam is highly collimated, yielding a field on the skin 54 mm in diameter. After positioning the patient, a superior angulation of 20 degrees and a posterior angulation of 15 degrees are easily set. A relatively long focus-to-film distance is used. Because of the angulation of the X-ray beam, only the bones of the cranium are superimposed over the joint, resulting in a sharp image of the mandibular condyle, fossa, and articular eminence.

The transcranial radiograph shows mainly the lateral part of the joint. It gives an impression of the condylar position within the mandibular fossa, the condylar dimensions (e.g., the condylar width reflected by the length of its oval projection), the depth of the mandibular fossa, the slope of the articular eminence, and the width of the joint space.

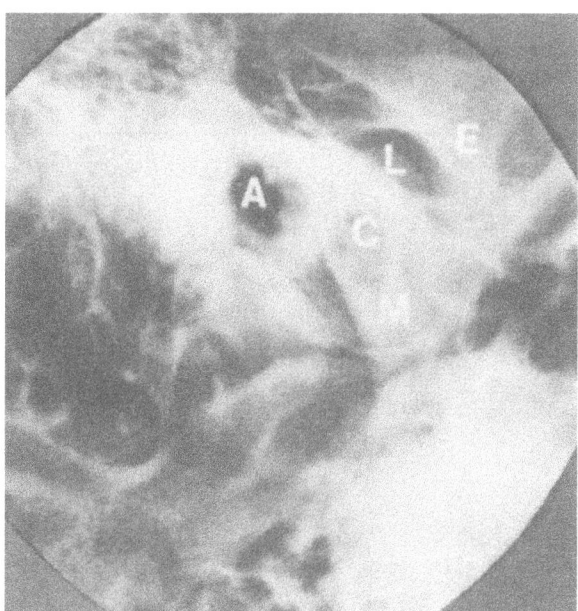

Figure 2.
Transcranial radiograph of
temporomandibular joint.
C = mandibular condyle,
L = lateral part of condyle,
M = medial part of condyle,
E = articular eminence,
A = auditory canal.

Transpharyngeal X-ray

The transpharyngeal X-ray (according to Parma, figure 3) is a contact exposure, made using an adapted dental X-ray tube. The open tube of the X-ray unit is placed against the skin over the mandibular notch, and the X-ray film cassette is placed against the skin on the other side of the head. The X-ray beam is highly collimated, yielding a field on the skin of only 16x30 mm. The central beam is directed towards the contralateral joint. Because of the short focus-to-skin distance (i.e., the ipsilateral joint is very close to the X-ray tube) and the divergence of the X-rays, the blurred projection of the ipsilateral joint is so vague that only the joint on the side of the film is visualized.

In order to standardize the transpharyngeal radiograph, a cephalostat attached to a dental chair was developed at our department, equipped for fixation of the head, attachment of the film cassette, and alignment of the X-ray tube. The patient is sitting in upright position in the dental chair and the radiograph is made with the patient's mouth maximally opened. Because of the standardization of head position and film and tube placement, this technique produces highly reproducible pictures.

The transpharyngeal radiograph offers an image of the temporomandibular joint, the condylar neck, the mandibular ramus, and part of the zygomatic area. Moreover, it provides an impression of joint mobility. It gives a detailed picture of the mandibular condyle. Deviations in shape, abnormalities of the bony structure, and irregularities in the cortical plate, i.e., all alterations that may be expected in the osteoarthrotic process, are well distinguishable. Degenerative

Figure 3.
Transpharyngeal radiograph
of temporomandibular joint.
C = mandibular condyle.
F = mandibular fossa.
E = articular eminence.
N = condylar neck.
R = mandibular ramus.

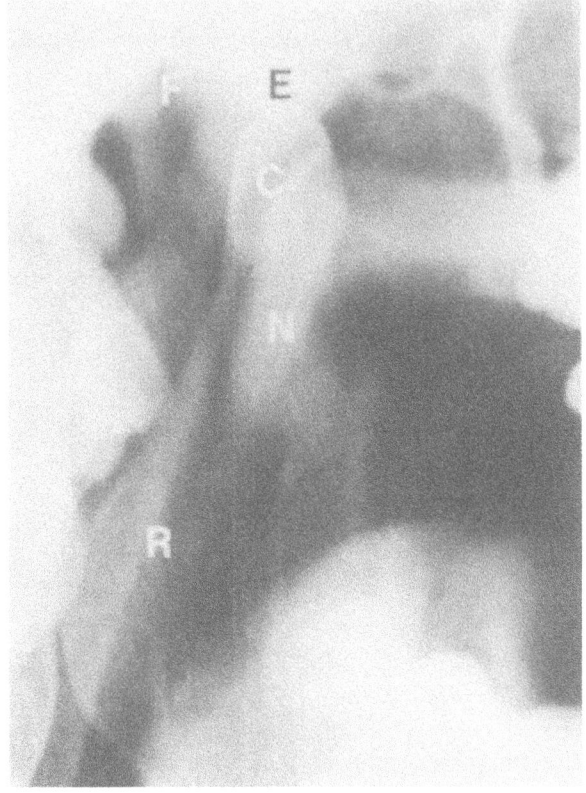

shortening of the condylar neck can be determined by comparing left and right transpharyngeal radiographs. The transpharyngeal X-ray is extremely useful in establishing a base-line documentation of a temporomandibular joint with osteoarthrotic symptoms. In repeated exposures, the progression of the disorder can be documented.

A frequently mentioned disadvantage of the transpharyngeal radiograph concerns the alleged high radiation dose to the patient. This objection to the technique is mainly based on the application of outdated dosimetric techniques (i.e., measurements of surface skin dose, now considered an invalid method for expression of radiation risk) and has been demonstrated to be irrelevant.[3]

Cephalometric X-rays

Cephalometric (lateral and antero-posterior) X-rays are used in specific cases only, e.g., suspected developmental disturbances such as condylar hyperplasia, or for documentation of acquired asymmetry due to shortening of the condylar neck as a result of late-stage osteoarthrosis.

Computerized tomography

Arthrography, computerized tomography, and magnetic resonance imaging are potentially useful for (indirect or direct) articular disc visualization. Extensive studies over a long period of time formerly established arthrography as the gold standard for disc imaging (figure 4). In the early 1980s, computerized tomography was described as a useful, non-invasive articular disc imaging technique by several investigators.[6-10] For the specific application of computerized tomography in temporomandibular joint diagnosis, a method was developed for direct sagittal scanning that proved to be superior to sagittal reconstruction from axial or coronal scans.[11] Reliability studies with regard to disc visualization showed major shortcomings of (direct sagittal) computerized tomography.[3] For imaging of soft tissue temporomandibular joint pathology, computerized tomography has been supplanted by magnetic resonance imaging.[3,12-14]

Nevertheless, (direct sagittal) computerized tomography offers excellent imaging of bony components of the joint, and has proved to be very useful, especially in differential diagnostic cases in which a more extended and complex disorder is suggested, but not clearly documented, on conventional radiographs.[14] Computerized tomography is superior to conventional radiographic methods, because with computerized tomography fine bone details can be visualized three-dimensionally without projectional limitations.[15] Furthermore, real shape and size of anatomical structures can be displayed.

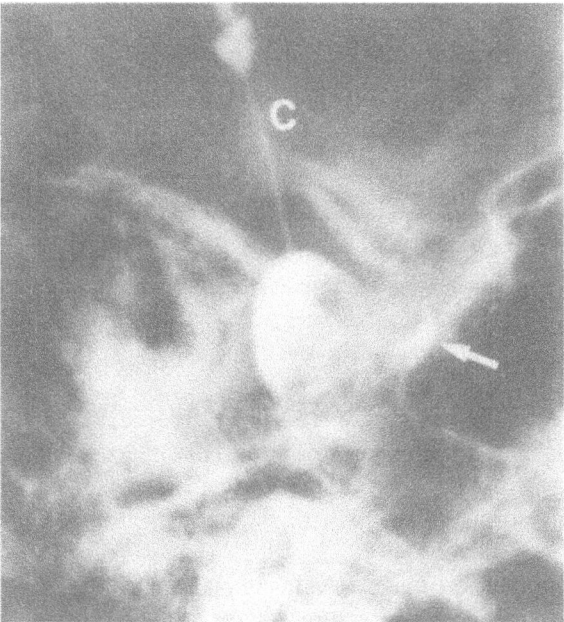

Figure 4.
Arthrogram of the temporomandibular joint.
Liquid contrast agent has
been injected into lower
joint space.

Direct sagittal computerized tomography is very effective in determining changes of condylar shape and position. Also, the glenoid fossa and articular eminence can be visualized. Moreover, osseous changes associated with whatever disease process, e.g., bone erosions, subchondral cysts, sclerosis, or remodeling, can be determined very effectively (figure 5).

The application of computerized tomography for differential diagnosis of temporomandibular disorders is not limited to arthropathies but can very well be expanded to non-articular disorders.[16] Its importance in the differential diagnosis of temporomandibular disorders has been illustrated in a series of cases of articular and non-articular disorders in which computerized tomography delivered invaluable diagnostic information that could not be derived from other imaging procedures.[14]

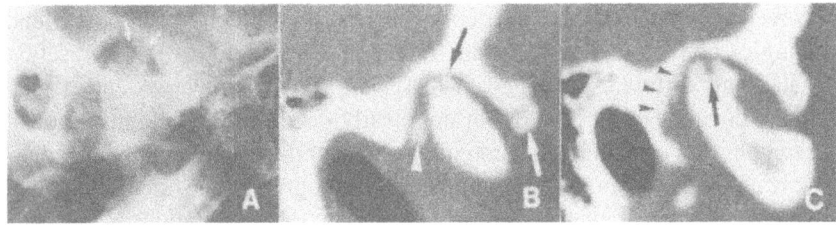

Figure 5.
Right temporomandibular joint, 58-year-old female: primary osteoarthrosis with severe degeneration, no obvious primary cause.
A. Transcranial: no joint space, osteolysis in lateral portion of condyle (arrows).
B. Direct sagittal CT, lateral portion: bony apposition on top of condyle (black arrow), on top of eminence (white arrow) and calcified loose body at posterior side of condyle (arrowhead).
C. Direct sagittal CT, midsagittal portion: subarticular cyst-like radiolucency on top of condyle (arrow), apposition of calcified material in posterior area of glenoid fossa (arrowheads).

Selected cases illustrating the value of computerized tomography in differential diagnosis

Multiple surgeries, especially without proper post-operative physical therapy, may end up in fibrous ankylosis in combination with osseous changes (figures 6–9). When preparing an arthroplasty for these cases, it is necessary to know where the bony changes and associated soft tissue changes can be expected during surgery.

Alloplastic implant materials (e.g., Proplast, Teflon, and Silastic) have been advocated as disc replacement material. Since it is known that extended tissue responses are induced by these materials, resulting in further joint damage, only temporary Silastic sheeting seems to be justified, and permanent alloplastic implant material should be avoided in temporomandibular joint surgery. Computerized tomography has a great potential in imaging implant material because of its specific density and homogeneous structure (figures 8 and 9).

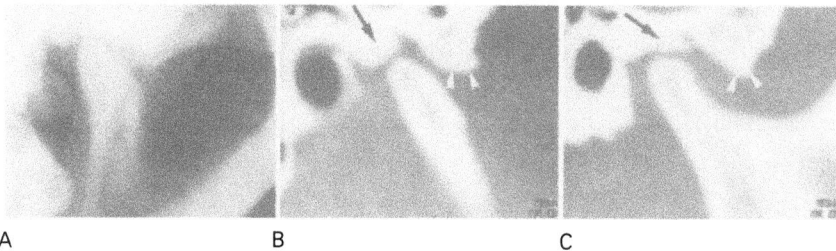

A   B   C

Figure 6. Left temporomandibular joint, 26-year-old female: secondary osteoarthrosis after trauma and multiple surgery.
A. Transpharyngeal: flattening of condyle, restricted translatory movement, no cortical lining of condyle, sclerosis of spongiosa, apposition of bone posteriorly in fossa.
B. Direct sagittal CT, lateral portion: apposition of bone posteriorly in glenoid fossa (arrow) and on top of eminence (arrowheads).
C. Direct sagittal CT, midsagittal portion: apposition of bone at roof of glenoid fossa (arrow) and on top of eminence (arrowheads).

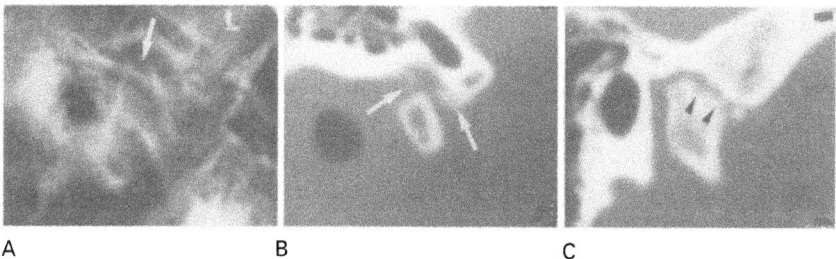

A   B   C

Figure 7. Left temporomandibular joint, 25-year-old female: bony/fibrous ankylosis after surgery.
A. Transcranial: osteolysis in lateral portion of the condyle (arrow), normal width of joint space, lack of bright imaging of joint space due to interposition of calcified tissue.
B. Direct sagittal CT, lateral portion: presence of calcified loose bodies in glenoid fossa (arrows).
C. Direct sagittal CT, medial portion: rudimental joint space, gigantiform condyle, irregular bony surface of condyle (arrowheads).

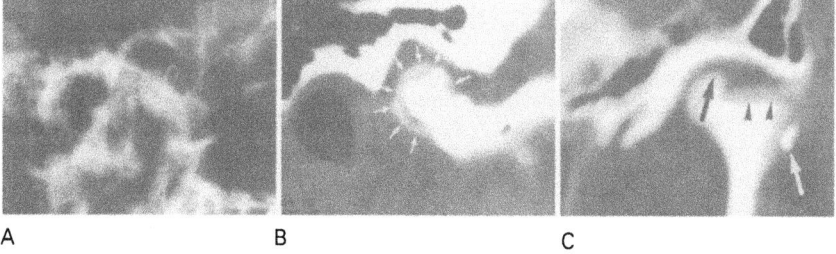

A   B   C

Figure 8. Right temporomandibular joint, 42-year-old female: fibrous ankylosis/secondary osteoarthrosis due to multiple surgeries including permanent Silastic sheeting.
A. Transcranial: metal wire in condylar area, widened joint space.
B. Sagittal CT, midsagittal portion: halo configuration around condyle (arrows), representing silastic sheeting, fixed to condyle.
C. Coronal CT: medial part of condyle shows original height (black arrow), midsagittal and lateral parts show features of partial high condylectomy with Silastic sheeting (arrowheads). Twisted metal ligature below lateral pole (white arrow).

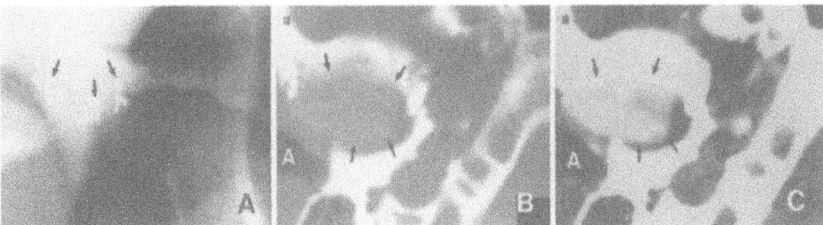

Figure 9. Right temporomandibular joint, 30-year-old female: fibrous ankylosis/secondary osteoarthrosis due to multiple surgeries including Silastic block implant.
A. Panoramic view: metal wiring in joint area (arrows). Loss of contour of condyle and eminence.
B. Axial CT, bone tissue window: mass of dense material in glenoid fossa, representing Silastic block implant (arrows). A = auditory canal.
C. Axial CT, soft tissue window: high contrast in glenoid fossa, representing Silastic block implant (arrows). A = auditory canal.

In craniofacial trauma diagnosis and treatment planning, computerized tomography is superior to conventional plain radiography and tomography in detecting fractures. Intra-capsular fractures, especially fractures of the medial pole of the condyle, cannot be easily detected on panoramic, transcranial, or transpharyngeal radiographs. Computerized tomography has the potential to discover them (figure 10).

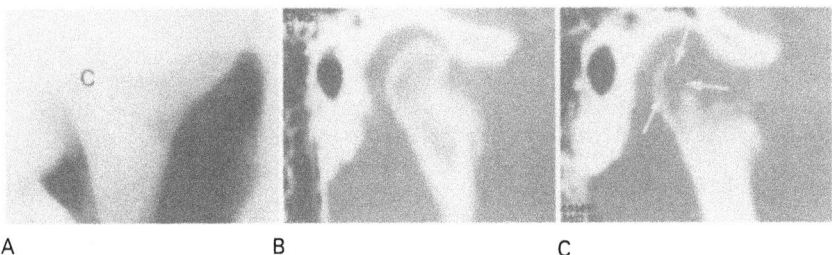

A   B   C

Figure 10. Right temporomandibular joint, 20-year-old male: intra-capsular fracture, destroyed medial pole of condyle.
A. Transpharyngeal: loss of clear contour of condyle (C), no translatory capacity, no fracture lines.
B. Direct sagittal CT, midsagittal portion: no features of fracture.
C. Direct sagittal CT, midsagittal portion (3.1 mm more medial than B): lysis of condylar bone due to fracture of medial portion of condyle (arrows).

In patients with ankylosis of the temporomandibular joint, plain radiographs and conventional tomography are of limited value because of problems of image distortion, loss of contour, and superimposition.[17] Bony ankylosis may be associated with extensive joint destruction and bone formation inside and outside the original contour of the joint. A mass of bone is the result, while the original joint structures cannot be properly recognized. Three-dimensional computerized tomography imaging is of great help in preparing a surgical

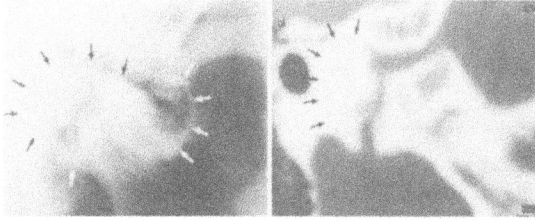

Figure 11. Left temporomandibular joint, 39-year-old male: bony/fibrous ankylosis.
A. Transpharyngeal: mass of bone (arrows) in joint region.
B. Direct sagittal CT, midsagittal portion: extended bone formation (arrows) in posterior portion of glenoid fossa, loss of normal condylar shape and size.

treatment plan. Direct sagittal computerized tomography reveals fine bony details (figure 11).

Crystal deposition diseases rarely occur in the temporomandibular joint. Gout and pseudogout have been reported.[18,19] The amount of deposed material can be considerable. Computerized tomography has the potential to display the calcified material inside the joint cavities (figure 12).

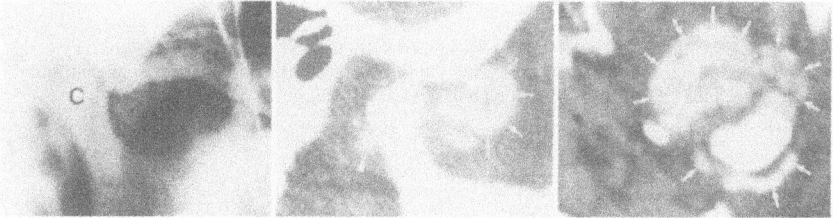

Figure 12. Left temporomandibular joint, 54-year-old female: calcium pyrophosphate dihydrate crystal deposition disease.
A. Panoramic view: normal contour of right condyle (C), no radiopaque material detectable around condyle.
B. Direct sagittal CT, midsagittal portion, soft tissue window: mass of calcified material in front of condyle (arrows) as well as behind condyle (arrowhead).
C. Axial CT, soft tissue window: extensive area of slightly calcified material (arrows) in front of condyle (C) and also medial, lateral, and posterior of condyle.

Generalized hypermobility of synovial joints is not related to temporomandibular joint osteoarthrosis.[20] It is still hypothesized, however, that hypermobility is a cause of juvenile osteoarthrosis and disc displacements in the temporomandibular joint.[4,20-22] Direct sagittal computerized tomography enables proper visualization of hypermobility associated with juvenile osteoarthrosis (figure 13).

Condylar hyperplasia is easily detectable, clinically as well as on conventional radiographs. Previously a case of condylar hyperplasia associated with

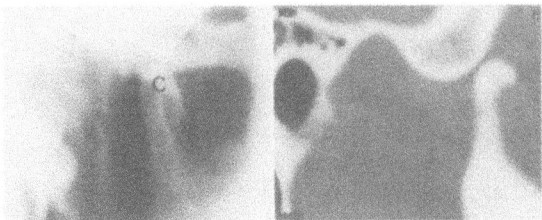

Figure 13. Right temporomandibular joint, 23-year-old female: secondary osteoarthrosis related to hypermobility.
A. Transpharyngeal: condyle in front of top of eminence (slight hypermobility), small condyle (C).
B. Direct sagittal CT, midsagittal portion: sclerosis of bone marrow, reduced size of condyle, slight anterior lipping, no extraordinary translatory capacity.

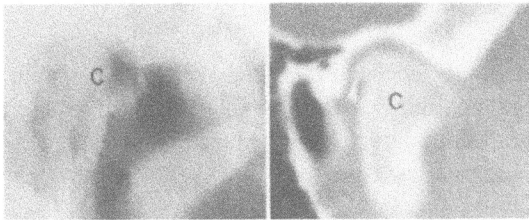

Figure 14. Right temporomandibular joint, 25-year-old male: condylar hyperplasia of right temporo-mandibular joint, active growing.
A. Transpharyngeal: unclear borderline of right gigantiform mandibular condyle (C).
B. Direct sagittal CT: clear-cut image of gigantiform mandibular condyle (C), note exophyte formation (arrowhead) at posterior side of condyle and flat eminence.

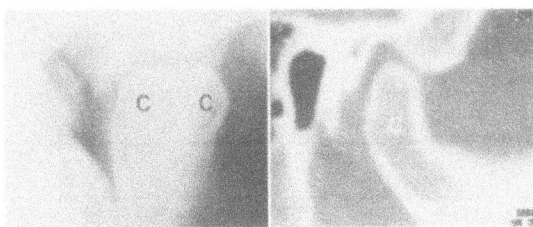

Figure 15. Left temporomandibular joint, 30-year-old male: overloading due to repeated minor trauma, pseudobifid condyle.
A. Transpharyngeal: bifid condyle (CC), normal range of motion.
B. Direct sagittal CT: midsagittal portion: normal shape and size of condyle (C), no bifid condyle.

synovial chondromatosis was reported in which the osteocartilaginous particles were not detectable by computerized tomography.[23] In figure 14, the bony details of the gigantiform condyle are shown by direct sagittal computerized tomography. Other puzzling phenomena on conventional radiographs can be solved with direct sagittal computerized tomography examination. A bifid condyle, displayed on the plain radiograph (figure 15A), may represent a large

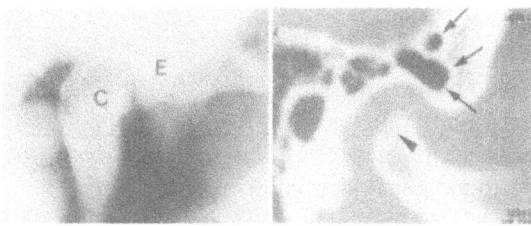

Figure 16. Left temporomandibular joint, 24-year-old female: secondary osteoarthrosis related to prior surgery. Pneumatic cavities in articular eminence.
A. Transpharyngeal: unclear cortical borderline of condyle (C) and eminence (E). No pneumatic cavities observable.
B. Direct sagittal CT: wide joint space, subarticular cyst (arrowhead), pneumatic cavities (arrowheads) in articular eminence.

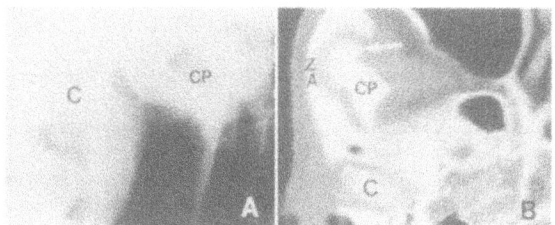

Figure 17. Right temporomandibular joint, 18-year-old male: pseudoankylosis due to impingement of osteoma at right mandibular coronoid process.
A. Panoramic view: vague image of bony extension of enlarged right coronoid process (CP).
B. Axial CT: mushroom-shaped bony structure (arrow) underneath zygomatic arch (ZA).
   C = condyle, CP = coronoid process.

condyle with the shape of a kidney (figure 15B). Pneumatic bone cavities of the articular eminence are an anatomical variation. Only when an eminectomy is planned, their presence has to be considered before surgery (figure 16).

Temporomandibular joint malignancy is rare. Metastases from malignant tumors elsewhere in the body, e.g., lung tumors, are occasionally found in the temporomandibular joint. Malignancies of the joint's surrounding tissues, e.g., parotid gland tumors, have to be taken into account in the differential diagnosis of a preauricular soft tissue swelling.[24-26] Parotid gland tumors may cause swelling in this region and may be associated with symptoms of dysfunction. Sialography may be helpful as well as computerized tomography, even for examination of soft-tissue pathology. Currently, however, magnetic resonance imaging has made a significant impact on parotid gland imaging.[27,28]

Extra-capsular pathology, e.g., osteoma or enlargement of the coronoid process, temporalis tendon fixation, or coronoid process impingement due to craniofacial trauma, may be a cause of restricted mouth opening (pseudoankylosis). Computerized tomography is extremely helpful in discovering the causative pathology (figure 17).

Conclusion

Computerized tomography is not indicated for routine temporomandibular joint imaging, but for imaging specific bony structures it is superior to plain films, tomography, and magnetic resonance imaging. The clarity and details permit a confident opinion with respect to the joint's normal or pathologic condition. Therefore, computerized tomography appears to be a proper imaging modality for temporomandibular joint differential diagnostic purposes.[29]

References

1 McNeill CH (ed). Craniomandibular disorders: guidelines for evaluation, diagnosis, and management. Chicago: Quintessence, 1990
2 Talley RL. Murphy GJ, Smith SD et al. Standards for the history, examination, diagnosis, and treatment of temporomandibular joint disorders (TMD): a position paper. J Craniomandibular Pract 1990; 8:60
3 van der Kuijl B. Temporomandibular Joint. Evaluation of imaging techniques. Thesis, University of Groningen, The Netherlands, 1992
4 Boering G. Arthrosis deformans van het kaakgewricht. Een klinisch en röntgenologisch onderzoek. Thesis, University of Groningen, The Netherlands, 1966
5 de Leeuw R. Temporomandibular Joint. A 30 year follow-up study of non-surgically treated temporomandibular joint osteoarthrosis and internal derangement. Thesis, University of Groningen, The Netherlands, 1994
6 Helms CA, Vogler JB, Morrish RB. Diagnosis by computed tomography of temporomandibular joint meniscus displacement. J Prosthet Dent 1984; 51:544
7 Manzione JV, Katzberg RW, Brodsky GL, et al. Internal derangements of the temporomandibular joint: diagnosis by direct sagittal computed tomography. Radiology 1984; 150:111
8 Sartoris DJ, Neumann CH, Riley RW. The temporomandibular joint: true sagittal computed tomography with meniscus visualization. Radiology 1984; 150:250
9 Manco LG, Messing SG, Busino LJ, et al. Internal derangements of the temporomandibular joint evaluated with direct sagittal CT: a prospective study. Radiology 1985; 157:407
10 Christiansen EL, Thompson JR, Zimmerman G, et al. Computed tomography of condylar and articular disk positions within the temporomandibular joint. Oral Surg Oral Med Oral Pathol 1987; 64:757
11 van der Kuijl B, Vencken LM, de Bont LGM, Boering G. Temporomandibular joint computed tomography: development of direct sagittal technique. J Prosthet Dent 1990; 64:709
12 Schellhas KP. Internal derangements of the temporomandibular joint: radiologic staging with clinical, surgical, and pathologic correlation. Magn Reson Imaging 1989; 7:495
13 Palacios E, Valvassori GE, Shannon M, Reed CF. Magnetic resonance of the temporomandibular joint. Stuttgart: Thieme, 1990
14 de Bont LGM, van der Kuijl B, Stegenga B, Vencken LM. Computed tomography in differential diagnosis of temporomandibular joint disorders. Int J Oral Maxillofac Surg 1993; 22:200
15 van der Kuijl B, Vencken LM, de Bont LGM, Boering G. Temporomandibular joint direct sagittal computed tomography: evaluation of imageprocessing modalities. J Prosthet Dent 1990; 64:589
16 Stegenga B, de Bont LGM, Boering G. A proposed classification of temporomandibular disorders based on synovial joint pathology. J Craniomandibular Pract 1989; 7:107
17 Solberg WK. Temporomandibular disorders: functional and radiological considerations. Br Dent J 1986; 160:195
18 Ballhaus S, Mees K, Vogl T. Infratemporaler Gichttophus eine seltene Differentialdiagnose zur primären Parotiserkrankung. Laryngol Rhinol Otol 1989; 68:638
19 Dijkgraaf LC, de Bont LGM, Liem RSB. Calcium pyrophosphate dihydrate crystal deposition disease of the temporomandibular joint. Report of a case. J Oral Maxillofac Surg 1992; 50:1003
20 Dijkstra PU, de Bont LGM, Stegenga B, Boering G. Temporomandibular joint osteoarthrosis and generalized joint hypermobility. J Craniomandibular Pract 1992; 10:221

21 Stegenga B, de Bont LGM, Boering G. Osteoarthrosis as the cause of craniomandibular pain and dysfunction. A unifying concept. J Oral Maxillofac Surg 1989; 47:249

22 Westling L. Temporomandibular joint dysfunction and systemic joint laxity. Thesis, University of Göteborg, Sweden; Swed Dent J 1992; suppl 81.

23 de Bont LGM, Blankestijn J, Panders AK, Vermey A. Unilateral condylar hyperplasia combined with synovial chondromatosis of the temporomandibular joint. Report of a case. Int J Oral Maxillofac Surg 1985; 13:32

24 Bavitz JB, Chewning LC. Malignant disease as temporomandibular joint dysfunction: review of the literature and report of case. J Am Dent Assoc 1990; 120:163

25 DelBalso AM, Sweeney AT, Kapur S. An unusual cause of facial trismus in a child: report of case. J Am Dent Assoc 1986; 112:207

26 Kaplan AS, Som PM, Lawson W. The coexistence of myofascial pain dysfunction and mucoepidermoid carcinoma of the parotid gland: report of case. J Am Dent Assoc 1986; 112:495

27 Freling NJM. MRI van parotistumoren. Een onderzoek naar de waarde van kernspinresonantietomografie bij 146 patiënten met een zwelling in de parotisloge. Thesis, University of Groningen, The Netherlands, 1991

28 Schaefer SD, Maravilla KR, Close LG, et al. Evaluation of NMR versus CT for parotid masses: a preliminary report. Laryngoscope 1985; 95:945

29 Salon JM. Computerassisted scanning of supracondylar fractures. Oral Surg Oral Med Oral Pathol 1990; 69:133

Management of Temporomandibular
Joint Degenerative Diseases
ed. by B. Stegenga & L.G.M. de Bont
© 1996 Birkhäuser Verlag Basel/Switzerland

The current role of magnetic resonance imaging in temporomandibular joint treatment planning

Quentin N. Anderson

HCMC Department of Medical Imaging, University of Minnesota, Minneapolis, Minnesota 55415-1829, USA

Summary: In this chapter, multiple-plane magnetic resonance imaging, disc cartilage magnetic resonance signal characteristics, and imaging characteristics of joint effusion and bone marrow signal parameters are discussed and illustrated.

Introduction

Over the past 70 years, medical imaging has significantly improved our ability to detect temporomandibular joint soft tissue and bone pathology.[1] The earliest work, i.e., transcranial views, depicted osseous abnormalities. The anatomic shortcomings of transcranial views, i.e., only lateral joint space visualization, were obviated when temporomandibular joint tomography was introduced. Tomography can image the entire lateral to medial joint surface. With the introduction of arthrography of the temporomandibular joint, the concept of disc position and joint function was introduced. This scientific concept attracted little attention until the early 1970s, when double-space arthrotomography was developed. Temporomandibular joint internal derangements could be detected and classified rather than assigned to pain-dysfunction syndromes. Computerized tomography of the temporomandibular joint evolved during the late 1970s and early 1980s. Bone pathology was accurately depicted; however, the detection of soft tissue (disc) pathology lacked sensitivity and specificity.

Magnetic resonance imaging was introduced in the 1980s. Its basic principles evolved from the biochemistry laboratories of the 1940s. In the late 1970s, the concept of tissue resonance was introduced, i.e., modulation of the external magnetic field within small tissue volumes. Selected relaxation sequences arising from specified volumes could be processed into distinct signal patterns. Currently, clinical magnetic resonance imaging reflects proton (H^+) density within a given tissue volume. High-energy phosphate imaging (spectroscopy) of muscle metabolism and functional brain imaging relative to joint function and motion are limited to research protocols.

There are no significant biologic side effects of magnetic resonance imaging. However, some precaution do need to be taken. The magnetic field can disable cardiac pacemakers, and metallic objects such as intracranial vascular clips and strategically placed metallic foreign bodies can be inadvertently distracted. Displacement of vascular clips can potentially create intracranial bleeding, and deflection of foreign bodies within the eye can affect vision. Dental fillings, braces, and joint prostheses are not affected by the magnetic field. X-ray imaging studies do not affect vascular clips or pacemakers, but they do rely on different tissue absorption of ionizing radiation. In addition, X-ray imaging of the disc requires percutaneous placement of contrast into the joint spaces. Magnetic resonance imaging, on the other hand, is non-invasive and utilizes a non-ionizing imaging technique. This, along with the physiologic principles of magnetic resonance imaging, makes it a very appealing modality.[1,2,3]

In this chapter, the following parameters of magnetic resonance imaging are discussed:

– multiple planes of imaging
– disc cartilage signal characteristics
– joint effusion
– bone marrow signal parameters.

Multiple planes of imaging

Sagittal and coronal planes

Multiplanar images can be derived from a single magnetic resonance imaging study. Most clinical studies utilize a spin echo technique, a high field strength magnet (1.5 tesla), thin section cuts (3 mm or less), small surface coils (FOV 16 cm or less), and multiple relaxation times (T1 and T2).[2,4]

Figure 1 shows a case with a Silastic joint implant and degenerative changes of the condyle. The condyle is flattened and elongated. The tomogram delineates sclerosis, flat contour of the condyle, and spur formation (figure 1A). Cortical bone is usually represented by a thin white pencil line of cortex, not the distorted contour and change in form as seen in this case.

The bone pattern on magnetic resonance images is twofold. Cortical bone has few protons, and thus registers as a dark signal on both T1 and T2 images. The marrow cavity of bone has a predominance of fatty tissue, a high proton content, and thus will be bright on T1 and show grey to low-signal intensity on T2 images. In this particular case, the low-signal intensity, irregular black cortical thickness of the condyle and mixed marrow patterns correlate with the sagittal tomogram. The smooth, concave contour of the condyle can be easily identified on sagittal and coronal planes of imaging (figure 1B and 1C). Sites of erosion and degenerative changes are easily identified. In our study groups coronal views have increased our detection of osteoarthrosis by 16%.

Magnetic resonance imaging may be of value in evaluating acute (figure 2) and healed (figure 3) mandibular fractures. The degree of medial rotation, angulation, and soft tissue injury can be evaluated in a non-invasive manner.

A

Figure 1.
A. Tomogram: flat contour of condyle and spur formation.
B. T1 sagittal MRI, closed position.
C. T1 coronal, closed position.
   Vertical arrow: bony erosive changes, osteoarthrosis.
   Arrowhead: residual Silastic in medial joint space.

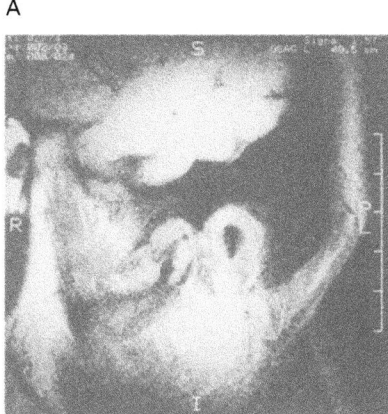

B

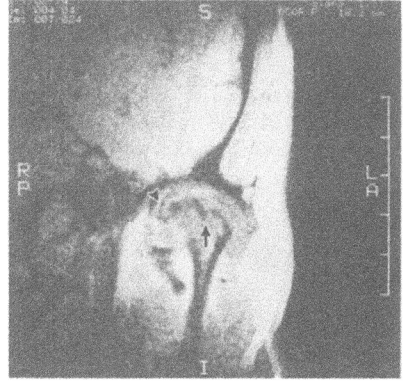

C

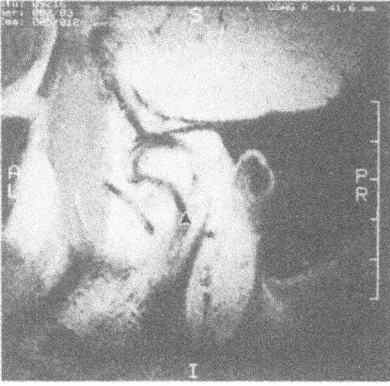

A

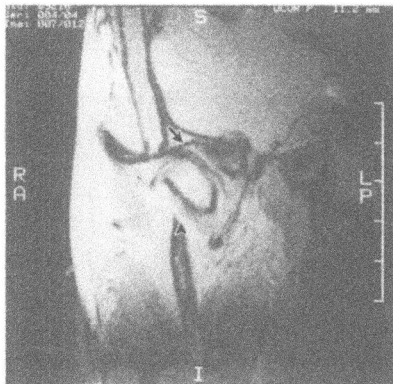

B

Figure 2.
A. T1 sagittal MRI, closed position. The arrowhead identifies the condylar neck fracture. The condylar head is rotated antero-medially due to the lateral pterygoid muscle attachment.
B. T1 coronal MRI, closed position. The arrowhead identifies the condylar neck fracture. The arrow identifies the medially rotated condylar head and disc.

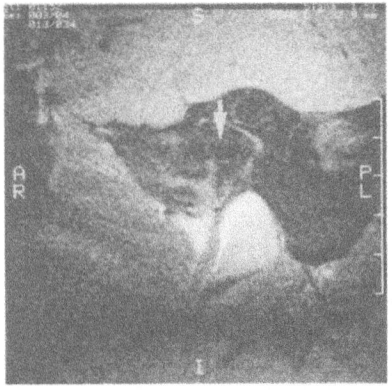

A

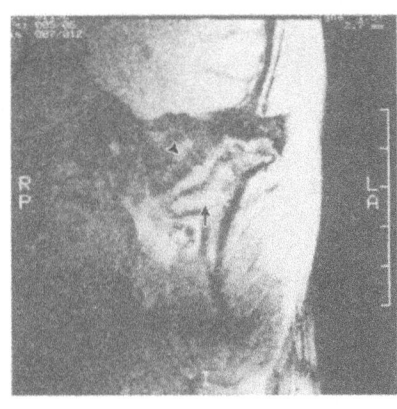

B

Figure 3.
A. T1 sagittal MRI, closed position.
   The arrow identifies the poorly outlined
   deformed contour of a healed condylar
   fracture.

B. T1 coronal MRI, closed position.
   The vertical arrow identifies the healed
   condylar fracture, medial inferior rotation of
   the condylar head. The arrowhead identifies
   the medial thickened residual disc.

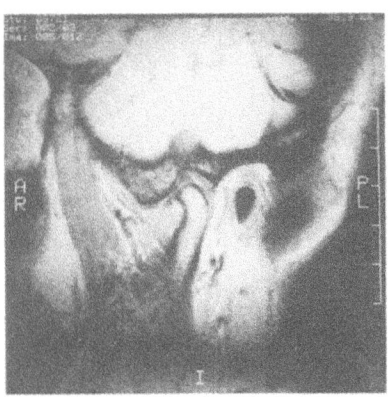

A

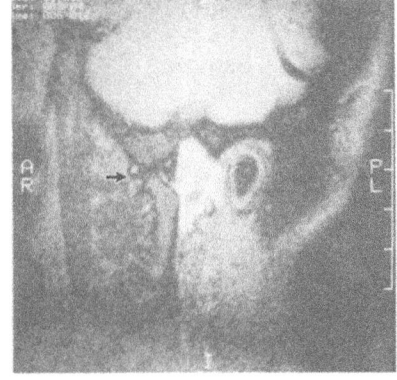

B

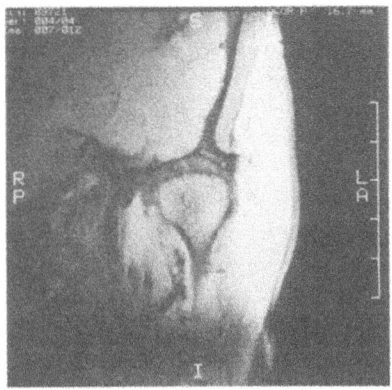

C

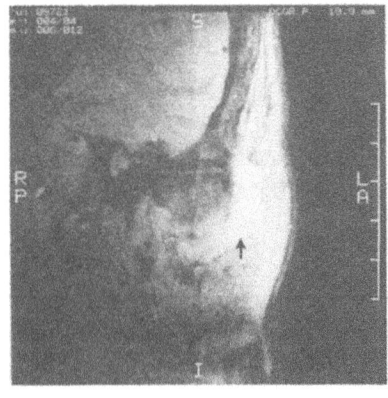

D

Figure 4.
A. T1 sagittal MRI, normal joint in closed position.
B. T2 sagittal MRI, open position.
   The arrow identifies fluid in the joint.
C. T1 coronal MRI, normal joint in closed position.

D. T2 coronal MRI, closed position.
   The arrow identifies polylobulated fluid,
   capsule pathology of rheumatoid arthritis.

Coronal images frequently provide the best view for assessing the extent of damage (figure 2B). This information is helpful in planning and evaluating surgical versus non-surgical therapy.

Figure 4 is a case of rheumatoid arthritis and illustrates the problem of detecting joint capsule pathology. The signal pattern of joint fluid on a T1 image is low to intermediate (dark); on T2 images the joint fluid registers a bright high-signal pattern (white). In this case of early rheumatoid involvement the polylobular capsular extensions and associated joint fluid are best demonstrated on coronal views (figure 4D). The sagittal views are essentially non-diagnostic and would underestimate the degree of soft tissue pathology.

Disc displacement occurs in the anteromedial direction in the majority of cases. In our institutional study groups, only a small percentage of displacements

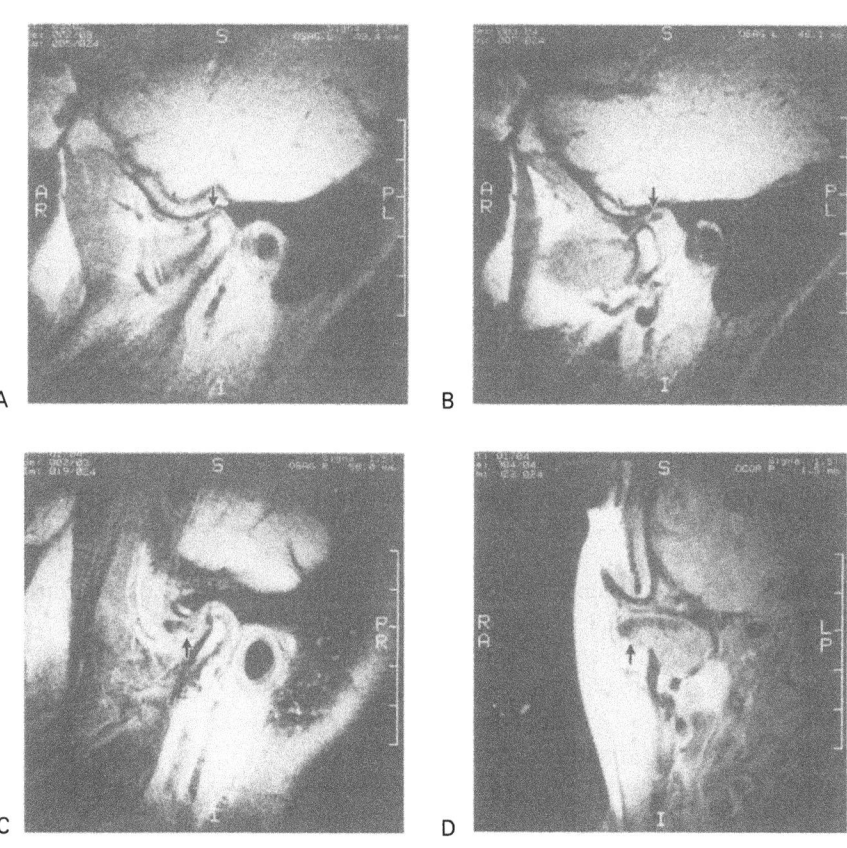

Figure 5.
A. T1 sagittal MRI, closed position.
   The arrow identifies that there is no disc in the joint space (empty fossa).
B. T1 sagittal MRI, open position.
   The arrow identifies a normal reduced disc position.
C. T1 sagittal MRI, closed position.
   The arrow identifies an anteriorly displaced, thickened disc.
D. T1 coronal MRI, closed position.
   The arrow identifies the lateral disc displacement (anterolateral disc position).

(approximately 2%) occur in the true lateral or medial direction. In the sagittal imaging plane medial or lateral disc displacement is often underestimated. The disc is not anatomically positioned between the condyle and glenoid fossa (the "empty fossa sign", figure 5A). In case studies of medial and lateral displacement the disc is most often thickened (figure 5C), and a small amount of joint fluid is usually present. Though joint fluid and increased disc size improve the detection rate of disc position, coronal views are indispensable (figure 5D). In one of our study groups, 12% of cases with disc rotation were either diagnosed or validated on coronal views. Thus we recommended that sagittal images be supplemented with coronal images for complete assessment of disc position.

Axial plane

In addition to sagittal and coronal imaging axial views can be made. This plane of imaging can be used to evaluate pathology of disc and bone or the maxillary sinuses, which may be another etiologic factor to consider in patients with atypical facial pain.

Signal characteristics of disc cartilage

Articular disc cartilage is composed of compact type I collagen with interposed elastic fibers and glycosaminoglycans. On both T1 and T2 weighted images the disc has a low to intermediate signal pattern. The cartilage is divided into zones or bands with the posterior band approximately 3 mm, the central zone approximately 1-2 mm, and the anterior band approximately 2 mm in thickness. The medial and lateral margins of the disc are firmly attached to the lateral and medial poles of the condyle. Anteriorly there is little discrete connection between the mandibular condyle and the disc, whereas posteriorly the fibers of the disc blend with the retrodiscal tissue. The retrodiscal tissue is composed of a loose network of collagen fibers, large elastic fibers, nerves, fat, and numerous blood vessels. The tissue is easily distracted and deformable in response to functional condylar motion (i.e., rotation, translation, and side-to-side motion).

In Figure 6 the condylar and temporal attachment of the retrodiscal tissue is illustrated. In figure 7A there is thickening of the retrodiscal tissue along with an anteriorly displaced reducing disc. The thickened attachments are a simple extension of the diffuse degenerative process within the disc. The T1 images of figure 7 also demonstrate increased signal intensity within the disc. Some investigators take this to indicate disc pathology representing structural failure. A preliminary review of our current study groups reveals that the greater majority of displaced discs, especially if there is associated hypertrophy (figure 7B), show a localized or uniform increase in signal intensity on T1 weighted images. This finding does not appear to have a positive correlation with overall integrity of the disc. These findings of increased T1 signal parallel the signal

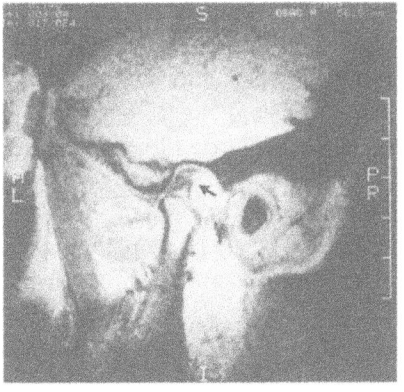

Figure 6.
A. T1 sagittal MRI, open position.
The arrow identifies the condylar and temporal posterior disc attachments.

B. T2 sagittal MRI, open position.
The arrow identifies the retrodiscal tissue, which is highlighted by the joint effusions.

patterns of medial and lateral knee cartilage, which have been classified relative to the signal intensity as grade I (low signal intensity) to grade III (high signal intensity). Grade I and grade III signal intensities are considered within normal limits. A grade III signal extends to the articular surface with some degree of architectural distortion. As such, simple presence of an increased signal within the cartilage does not uniformly signify pathology.[5,6]

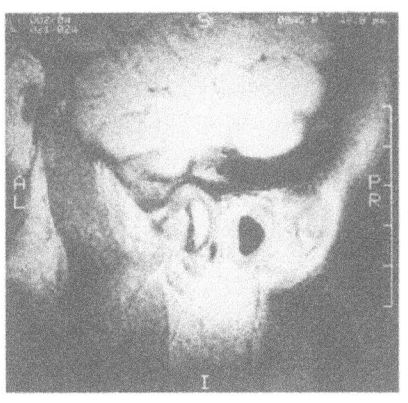
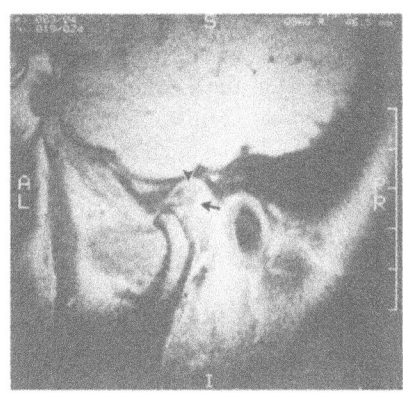

Figure 7.
A. T1 sagittal MRI, closed position.
The disc is anteriorly displaced and thickened.
B. T1 sagittal MRI, open position.
The posterior arrow identifies the thickened condylar and temporal attachments of the disc (retrodiscal tissue). The vertical arrowhead identifies the areas of increased signal with the posterior disc. This increased signal is a frequent finding in disc hypertrophy and is of no predictive value (disc variability).

We have recently analyzed 27 cases pre- and post-discoplasty. Pre-operatively, 30% of the discs had slight or intermediate increase in signal intensity. Twenty-two of the 27 cases had successful surgical repositioning. Analysis of the five failures revealed no disproportionate increase in signal intensity on either pre-operative or post-operative images. In addition, three of the 22 successful cases had significant disc hypertrophy, which required surgical recontouring of the disc. The magnetic resonance imaging pattern between contoured and non-contoured cases was the same. The study is ongoing with 7-12 month follow-up. To date, post-surgical outcomes have not correlated with increased disc signal.

Another consideration with regard to increase in T1 signal intensity relates to the anatomic relationships of the temporomandibular joint. The temporomandibular joint is anatomically positioned at 55 degrees to the magnetic field and can undergo a signal conversion such that on a T1 weighted image increased signal intensity is registered. The disc cartilage is positioned at 55 degrees; thus, any increase in signal may simply be attributed to a combination of factors (i.e., anatomic variant as well as this "magic angle effect").[7]

Joint effusion

Detecting joint effusion prior to magnetic resonance imaging was difficult. In the author's personal experience of several thousand arthrograms, it was a rarity to aspirate a significant amount of joint fluid. Several recent papers have supported the idea that the amount of joint fluid can be correlated with the patient's symptomatology. In our study groups this has not proven to be useful. This lack of correlation is not unexpected. In the recent past, we did joint fluid analysis of 22 consecutive cases of internal derangement. We analyzed the aspirated fluid for biochemical factors, including substance P, and found no correlation between symptomatology, stage of internal derangement, or level of substance P. Our final conclusion was that the mechanical effect of internal derangement does not correlate with the amount of biochemical mediators in the joint fluid.

Joint effusions are common. Seventy-five percent of our cases with internal derangements have a joint effusion. In addition, fluid can also be detected in 15-20% of asymptomatic normals.

Bone marrow signal intensity

Alterations of the bone marrow pattern (i.e., dark T1 and bright T2, reflecting edema) have lead some investigators to propose a theory that this is diagnostic of avascular necrosis. Avascular necrosis is a multi-factorial dysfunction of microcirculation. The pathophysiology relates to occlusive substances within the vessel lumen, abnormalities of the vessel wall, or abnormalities within

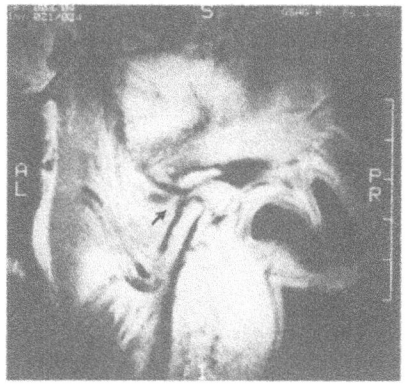
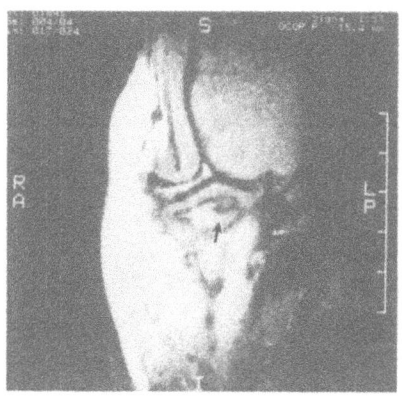

A   B

Figure 8.

A. T1 sagittal MRI, open position.
   The arrow identifies the non-reduced anterior
   disc position with degenerative changes in the
   condyle.

B. T1 coronal MRI, closed position.
   The arrow identifies a subchondral arc of low
   signal intensity (crescent sign).

surrounding marrow space. It is interesting to note that avascular necrosis only occurs in fatty marrow. This may relate to a difference in microcirculation (fatty marrow versus hemopoietic marrow).

The nutrient and periosteal blood supply to the condyle is abundant. Nearly every vessel within 2 cm of the temporomandibular joint supplies a vascular branch, and there are variable and numerous routes of collateral blood flow. There are no valid studies that substantiate the theory that medial disk displacement compromises the vascular supply and is a cause of avascular necrosis in the condyle.[8]

Figure 8 illustrates presumptive findings of avascular necrosis. On the T1 weighted image there is a very slight decrease in signal intensity (figure 8A); the T2 weighted images show a slight increase in signal intensity. Coronal views reveal a low signal, somewhat crescent-shaped deformity in the subarticular region of the mid-condyle (figure 8B). The patient did have a closed-lock and was appropriately treated with interventional surgery.

In our study groups, the findings of a decreased T1 and slightly increased T2 signal occurs in a very small percentage of cases (1% or less). The findings are non-specific and can be found in transient osteoporosis, stress fracture, osteomyelitis, marrow infiltration pattern, and early phase avascular necrosis. Without supportive documentation or scientific analysis there is little evidence to support aggressive interventional therapy.

Figure 9 illustrates a diminished bone marrow signal ("black condyle"). The lack of marrow signal intensity, i.e., absence of fat within the marrow space, does not reflect the overall integrity of the condyle. This simply means that the fatty marrow has been replaced, usually with hemopoietic or fibrous material. We do not have a magnetic resonance signal pattern for an osteoblast or

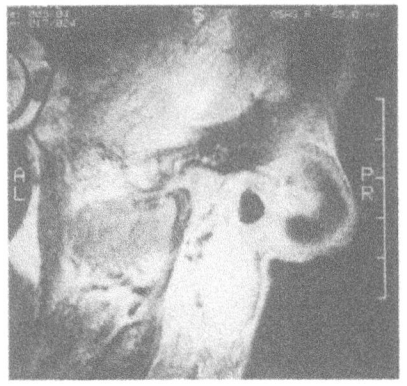
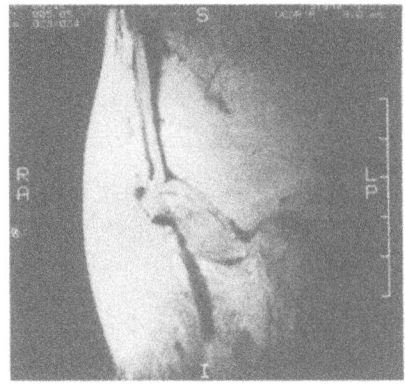

A   B

Figure 9.

A. T1 sagittal MRI, open position.
   The marrow signal in the condyle is absent
   (fatty marrow replacement). There is also an
   anterior disc displacement.

B. T1 coronal MRI, closed position.
   The marrow signal in the condyle is absent
   (fatty marrow). The load stress integrity of
   bone is not affected by fatty marrow replacement.

osteoclast. Black condyles occur in 1-2% of our study cases. They are most often associated with disc displacement.[9,10,11]

In orthopedics, long-bone fractures of the upper and lower extremities are treated by placing metallic rods in the marrow cavity of long bones. This often requires that the bone marrow space be anatomically removed (i.e., a surgically created black marrow pattern). Treating fracture cases in this fashion does not significantly alter the rate of success of bone repair.

Figure 10 illustrates an iatrogenic causality for decreased marrow signal, i.e., granulomatous response from Proplast allograft. The diminished signal pattern simply reflects fibrosis secondary to the giant cell reaction. Magnetic resonance imaging is useful in identifying and quantifying the degree of granulomatous response but has no predictive value relative to the viability of the condyle or glenoid fossa.

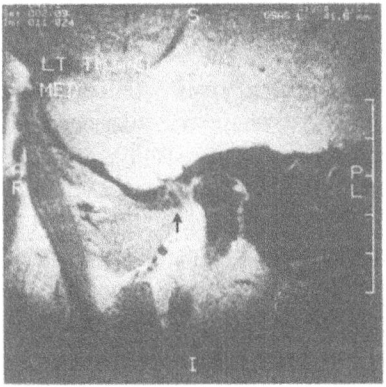

Figure 10.
T1 weighted sagittal MRI, closed position.
The arrow identifies the condyle and joint
space which have been replaced by giant cell
reaction from proplast.

Conclusion

There are multiple approaches to temporomandibular joint imaging. Magnetic resonance imaging studies in multiplanar format are standard at our institution. We still do concurrent X-ray tomography for validation of osseous abnormalities. Rapid acquisition magnetic resonance imaging techniques shorten imaging time and can be used to evaluate joint motion. These features may enhance patients' acceptance and throughput but have not perceptively changed our accuracy in detecting internal derangement. Late-stage disc perforations cannot be identified on magnetic resonance images. This can only be done with contrast injection into the lower joint space.

The future challenge of outcome analysis (cost/benefit) can only be answered with appropriate medical imaging. Multiplanar magnetic resonance imaging exams are accurate, non-invasive, and reproducible.

References

1 Roberts D, Pelligrew J, Ram C. A review of radiologic techniques to evaluate the temporomandibular joint. I. Conventional radiography. Anesth Progr 1984; 31:197
2 Katzberg RW, Westesson PL. Diagnosis of the temporomandibular joint. Philadelphia: Saunders, 1993
3 Christiansen EL. Temporomandibular joint X-ray computed tomography. Methodology and clinical applications. Thesis, Karolinska Institutet Stockholm, Sweden, 1988
4 Roberts D, Schenck J, Joseph P. Magnetic resonance imaging of the temporomandibular joint meniscus. Radiology 1985; 154:829
5 Mink JH. MRI imaging of the musculoskeletal system. New York: Raven Press, 1990
6 Scapino R. Histopathology associated with malposition of the human temporomandibular joint disc. Oral Surg Oral Med Oral Pathol 1983; 55:382
7 Ericsson SJ. The "magic angle" effect: background physics and clinical relevance. Radiology 1993; 188:23
8 Takagi R. Angiography of the temporomandibular joint. Oral Surg Oral Med Oral Pathol 1994; 78:539
9 Roberts D. Efficacy of MRI for clinical diagnosis of TMJ pathology: preliminary results. J Dent Res 1989; 68:761
10 Lang P. Avascular necrosis of the femoral head: high-field-strength MR imaging with histologic correlation. Radiology 1988; 169:517
11 Colwell CW. The controversy of core decompression of the femoral head for osteonecrosis. Arthr Rheum 1989; 32:797

Management of Temporomandibular
Joint Degenerative Diseases
ed. by B. Stegenga & L.G.M. de Bont
© 1996 Birkhäuser Verlag Basel/Switzerland

Current role of diagnostic arthroscopy in temporomandibular joint treatment planning

Ken-Ichiro Murakami and Natsuki Segami

Department of Oral and Maxillofacial Surgery, Faculty of Medicine, Kyoto University Hospital, Japan

Summary: Diagnostic arthroscopy should be considered as a refinement of clinical diagnosis with regard to specific joint tissue abnormalities, such as synovitis and adhesion formation, and their severity. This method is also advised prior to scheduled surgery, to record intra-articular findings and relate them to clinical signs and symptoms. In the future, diagnostic arthroscopy could be valuable in the detection of early pathologic changes of articular cartilage, especially when combined with chemical joint fluid analysis.

Introduction

In the past decade, arthroscopy has been advanced as a diagnostic and surgical tool in the field of temporomandibular disorders. Direct inspection of the joint space has widened our knowledge and influenced our perspective with regard to articular pathophysiology.

The clinical application of temporomandibular joint arthroscopy was first reported by Ohnishi.[1] Murakami, and Holmlund et al. independently provided data with regard to diagnostic arthroscopy of the temporomandibular joint.[2-5] Arthroscopic lysis and lavage of the upper joint cavity in patients with closed-lock was thereafter reported by Sanders.[6]

The aim of this chapter is to provide a description of arthroscopic anatomy and diagnostic examination, and to discuss the significance of diagnostic procedures in temporomandibular joint degenerative diseases.

Arthroscopic anatomy

Anatomical landmarks of importance for identification and interpretation of intra-articular pathologic changes include the position and condition of the articular disc, the capsule, the retrodiscal tissue, and the articular surfaces of eminence and condylar head. The upper joint compartment is routinely inspected during diagnostic arthroscopy, while the lower joint space is inspected in selected cases or when there is rupture or perforation of the disc or its attachment. In order to ensure a systematic inspection, it is important to recognize the structures that are visualized during the arthroscopic procedure.

Figure 1.
A. Intra-articular systematic
   observation of the upper
   joint compartment by the
   inferolateral approach.
   1: upper posterior synovial
      pouch;
   2: upper anterior synovial
      recess;
   3: intermediate space;
   (Au) auditory canal;
   (Ll) lateral ligament;
   (Lt) lateral pterygoid
   muscle;
   (Re) retrodiscal tissue;
   (St) superficial temporal
   artery and vein.

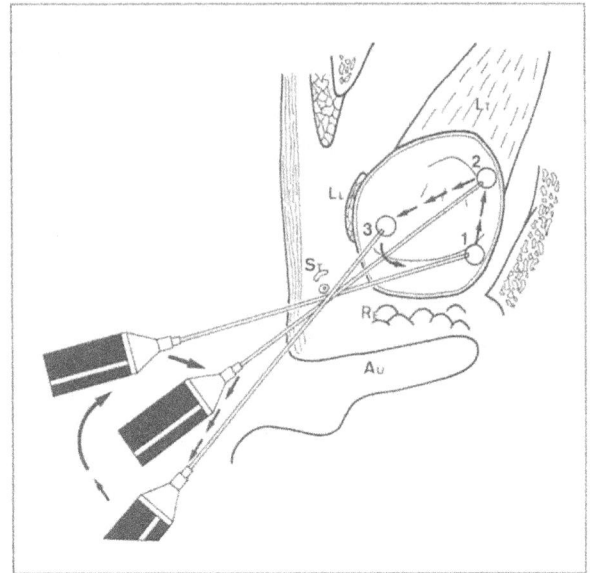

B. Arthroscopic view of the
   upper posterior synovial
   pouch (right temporo-
   mandibular joint).
   (P) retrodiscal tissue;
   (M) medial capsule;
   (F) mandibular fossa.

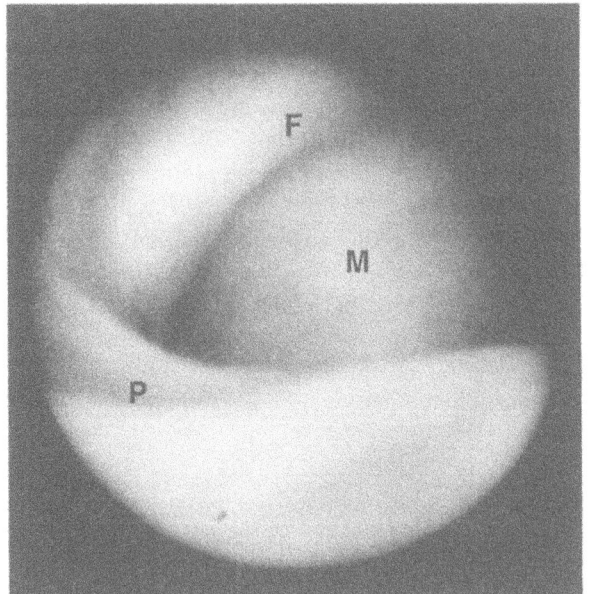

Since anatomic descriptions have been reported in detail in the literature,[2,4] we will briefly describe only the most important landmarks.

The conventional approach to systematic arthroscopic examination of the upper joint cavity is shown in figure 1. In order to decide whether the upper or lower joint space is to be inspected, the jaw is manipulated anteriorly by the assisting surgeon. A step-by-step examination of the upper compartment is

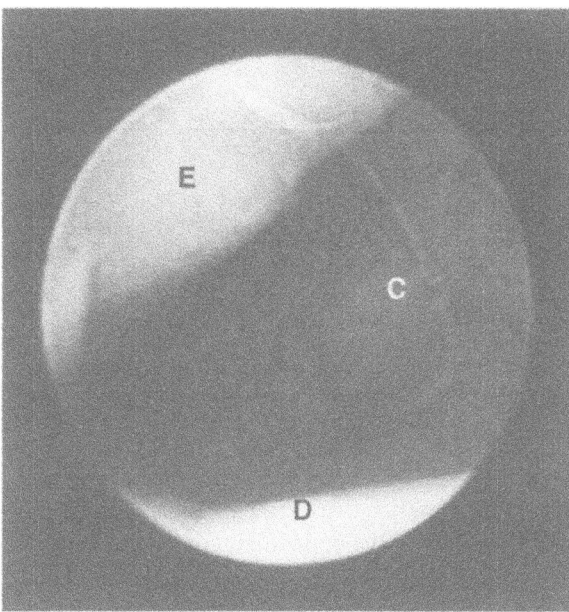

Figure 2.
Arthroscopic view of the upper anterior synovial recess (right temporomandibular joint).
(E) articular eminence peak; (D) surface of anterior band of the disc; (C) anterior limit of capsule.

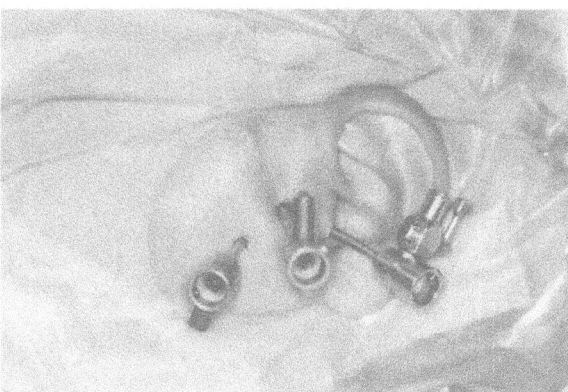

Figure 3A
Triple puncture (anterolateral, inferolateral, endaural) to upper joint compartment.

carried out from the anterior pouch to the intermediate space. Recognition of the anterior pouch is important to identify the anterior limit of the joint compartment and the lateral capsule (figure 2). A more extensive view is achieved by additional punctures at the anterior recess and via the endaural approach (figure 3A). In order to examine the lower joint compartment, usage of an ultra-thin arthroscope is advisable. Puncture is carried out towards the posterior surface of the mandibular condyle, after which the fine cannula is inserted into the posterior recess of the lower joint space (figure 3B). Further technical aspects are presented in the literature.[8]

Most commonly, diagnostic arthroscopy is performed under general anesthesia to assess or confirm the existing pathology prior to scheduled arthroscopic or open joint surgery. Diagnostic arthroscopy can also be carried out

Figure 3B
Arthroscopic view of
lower joint compartment
with ultra-thin arthroscope.
(C) condylar head;
(D) disc lower surface;
(PA) synovial surface of
retrodiscal tissue;
(AR) anterior synovial
pouch.

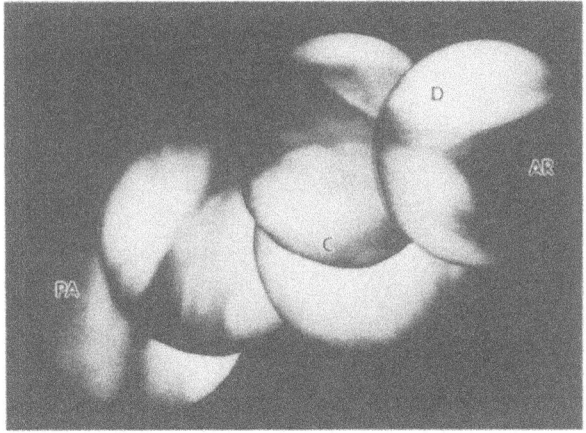

under local anesthesia with or without sedation in the outpatient clinic. The aim
is to inspect the intracapsular condition of the upper joint compartment. It can
also be performed in conjunction with arthrocentesis or pumping manipulation.
The step cannulation technique with the ultra-thin needle arthroscope is helpful
for safe and reliable puncture (figure 4).

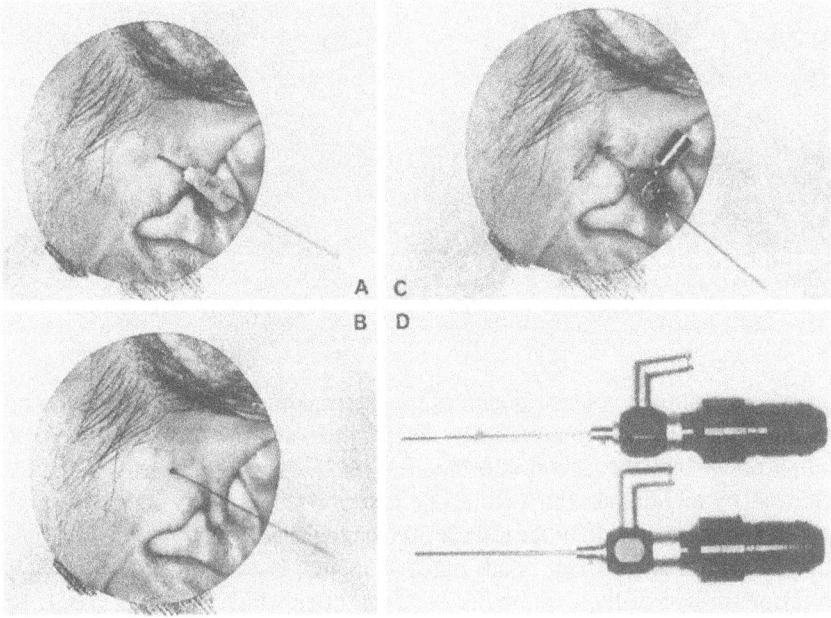

Figure 4.
Outpatient clinic arthroscopy.
A. Insertion of thin mandril through 21 gauge
   needle.
B. Needle removed, mandril left in joint space.

C. 1.3 mm canula inserted.
D. Ultra-thin arthroscopes (0.9 mm and 1.2 mm
   in diameter).

Diagnostic accuracy

The diagnostic accuracy of upper compartment arthroscopy has been investigated in human cadaver studies.[4,9,10] Holmlund et al. reported accuracies of 100% for osteoarthrosis and 57% for remodeling.[4] Liedberg et al. described the method to have low sensitivity (ranging from 0.21 to 0.67) and high specificity (ranging from 0.93 to 1.00).[9] The variation in sensitivity and specificity was related to the area of the joint being visualized. Bibb et al. reported abnormal soft tissue structure which became apparent after dissection and had not been discovered by neither tomography, arthrography, nor arthroscopy.[10] Each diagnostic modality appears to have its own advantages and disadvantages. Kondoh and Westesson assessed the diagnostic accuracy of lower joint compartment arthroscopy[8] and reported results accuracy comparable to that for upper compartment arthroscopy (57%).

Arthroscopy is not an appropriate screening tool for temporomandibular disorders due to its surgical morbidity. Its primary application is, therefore, to refine the clinical diagnosis with regard to specific tissue abnormalities and their severity.

Arthroscopic pathology

Synovitis (figure 5)

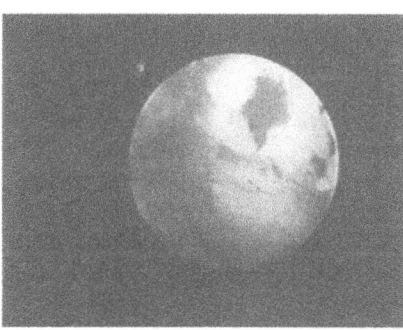

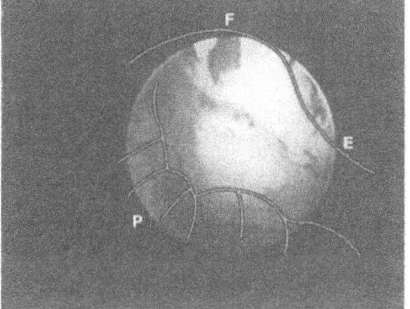

Figure 5.
Synovitis in upper posterior synovial pouch (right temporomandibular joint).
(F) fossa; (E) articular eminence; (P) retrodiscal tissue.

Table 1. Arthroscopy-based synovitis-index of Holmlund and Hellsing (1988)

Stage	Characteristics
SYN 0	Normal pale, almost translucent, synovial lining with a fine network of anastomosing small blood vessels
SYN I	Localized area with increased vascularity and capillary hyperaemia. Contact bleeding may occur during arthroscopy
SYN II	Generalized capillary hyperaemia, effusion, and debris. Arthroscopic examination is possible after irrigation of the joint cavity.

Holmlund et al. reported a significant correlation between joint pain and synovitis, using a three-level arthroscopic staging of synovitis (table 1).[5] Restricted opening and crepitus appear to correlate with the presence of osteoarthrosis.[5] Murakami et al. reported a positive correlation between pain during chewing and the presence of synovitis.[11] The limitation of these results is the subjective method of rating synovitis. A validated grading system for synovitis remains to be established.

Arthroscopic assessment of synovitis has been compared with histopathologic findings by Merrill et al. in 67 consecutive cases,[12] and by Holmlund et al. in 23 patients (25 joints).[13] Using the histologic findings as a gold standard, arthroscopic diagnosis of synovitis was reported to be highly accurate (sensitivity 1.0 and 0.94, specificity 0.89 and 0.86, respectively).

Quinn and Bazan reported their arthroscopic index of acute synovitis to correlate well with the level of prostaglandin E_2 and leukotrien B_4 in the synovial fluid of 19 painful temporomandibular joints[14]. On the other hand, Holmlund et al. did not find a significant correlation between several neuropeptides in the synovial fluid of 19 temporomandibular joints and clinical signs or symptoms[15].

The presence of synovitis is apparently related to the presence of arthralgia. Inflammatory mediators are believed to release enzymes, such as metalloproteases, which induce cartilage breakdown and joint degeneration. Therefore, it is important to identify the presence and severity of synovitis in joints with osteoarthrosis and internal derangements.

Fibrous adhesions (figure 6)

It has been suggested that adhesions contribute to joint locking.[6,16] Kaminishi and Davis described several types of adhesions.[17] Murakami et al. surveyed 68 consecutive temporomandibular joints in 56 patients and found a high incidence of adhesions (62 out of 68 joints). In a subset of 28 patients, the clinical signs were compared with the extent and distribution of adhesions. Pain and subjective jaw dysfunction were only weakly correlated with adhesions. A weak but statistically significant correlation was found between the interincisal

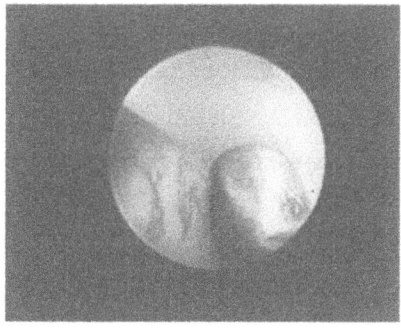

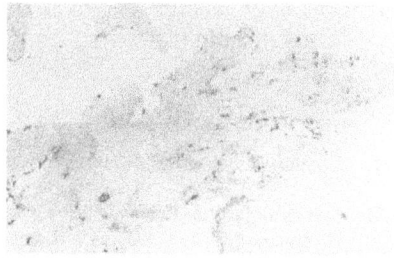

B

Figure 6.
A. Fibrous pseudo-wall adhesions at upper anterior synovial recess (right temporomandibular joint).
B. Histologic view of removed pseudo-wall adhesion, showing fibrous tissue with partly hyalinized degeneration.

A

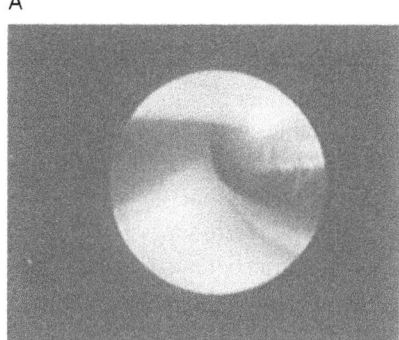

opening and the presence of adhesions.[18] It was concluded that, although adhesions probably alter joint mobility, there is little contribution of adhesions to temporomandibular joint pain and dysfunction.

Criteria for scoring the extent of adhesions are not well established, and a correlation between their histologic appearance (figure 6B) and clinical signs and symptoms has not been established. Reproducible rating of adhesions is, however, very difficult.

Degenerative alterations

In a study of 49 joint specimens, Holmlund and Hellsing reported 100% agreement between osteoarthrotic changes as observed by arthroscopic inspection and the corresponding dissection.[4] Based on arthroscopic observations, they distinguished three stages of osteoarthrosis (table 2). In another study, they showed that osteoarthrotic changes are frequently associated with synovitis.[19] In a study of 55 patients, the authors reported a statistically significant correlation between crepitus and advanced osteoarthrotic changes as observed arthroscopically, as well as between crepitus and disc perforation. A negative correlation was present between reciprocal clicking and arthroscopically determined osteoarthrotic changes.[5] From these studies it appears that advanced osteoarthrosis can be reliably detected by arthroscopic examination. However,

Table 2. Arthroscopy-based osteoarthrosis-index of Holmlund and Hellsing (1988)

Stage	Characteristics
OA 0	Smooth, glossy white-to-yellow surfaces of fibrocartilage and disc
OA I	Localized areas of superficial fibrillation of fibrocartilage and disc
OA II	One or more of the following features: (1) pronounced fibrillation of fibrocartilage and disc (2) exposure of subchondral bone (3) eburnation (4) disc perforation

these changes (with the exception of the detection of synovitis) can also be detected by less invasive procedures, such as conventional radiography.

Chondromalacia is not radiographically detectable, yet it can be detected by arthroscopic examination. Based on arthroscopic observations and the corresponding orthopedic literature, Quinn distinguished four stages of temporomandibular joint chondromalacia, i.e., softening, furrowing, fibrillation and ulceration, and crater formation with subchondral bone exposure.[20] He speculated that probable causes of pain in joints with chondromalacia include friction, compression and impingement of degenerated articular cartilage, and secondary synovitis. Unfortunately, at present Quinn's suggested classification and his hypothesis regarding associated pain mechanisms have not yet been validated. In our prospective comparative study, the loss of continuity of the contour of the articular eminence as observed on magnetic resonance images could not accurately be correlated with arthroscopic findings of chondromalacia (table 3).

In a study of 25 temporomandibular joints in 20 patients, Israel et al. showed that synovial fluid aspirated from joints with arthroscopically demonstrated osteoarthrosis contained higher levels of keratan sulphate than did fluid from joints without evidence of osteoarthrosis.[21] Further validation of the pathologic characteristics of chondromalacia and their relationship with clinical signs and symptoms is necessary.

Table 3. Comparison between magnetic resonance imaging (MRI) and arthroscopic findings of chondromalacia in 20 temporomandibular joints (14 patients)

	Arthroscopic findings	
	positive**	negative
MRI findings		
positive*	9	4
negative	9	8

* positive MRI findings represent irregularity and/or loss of continuity of the articular eminence contour
** positive arthroscopic findings of chondromalacia stage III and IV

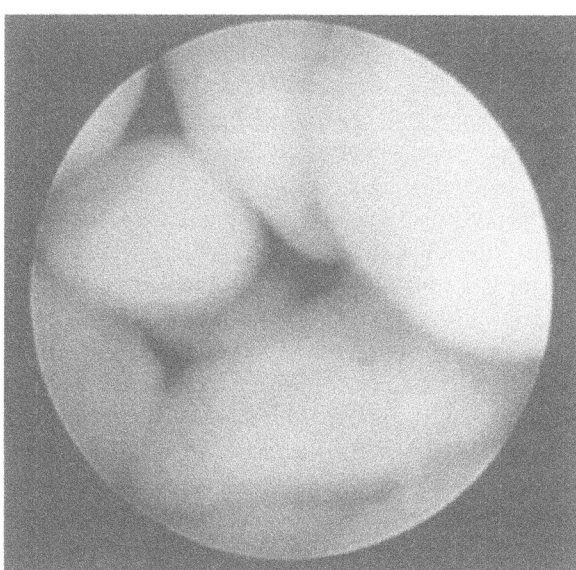

Figure 7.
Arthroscopic view in synovial chondromatosis.

Arthroscopic biopsy

Due to the lack of a device for taking core biopsy from the cartilaginous-osseous component of the temporomandibular joint, currently histopathologic evaluation is limited to arthroscopically obtained soft tissue and debridement material. Evaluating temporomandibular joint degenerative diseases by arthroscopic biopsy procedures is a major future challenge.

Arthroscopically visualized moderate to severe synovitis has been shown to correlate with histologic evidence of synovitis from arthroscopic biopsy specimens of inflamed synovial tissue.[12–13] However, the relationship between arthroscopically visualized mild synovitis and histologic evidence was not clear.

Rheumatoid arthritis may be well diagnosed based on arthroscopic biopsy material,[22] although further studies are necessary for grading the arthroscopic changes associated with rheumatoid arthritis.

The presence of numerous loose bodies in the joint space strongly suggests the diagnosis of synovial chondromatosis (figure 7), which can be confirmed by histologic evidence of cartilaginous nodules and cloned chondrocytes with hyperchromatic nuclei.

Diagnostic arthroscopy: indications and contra-indications

According to the position paper of the American Association of Oral and Maxillofacial Surgeons, diagnostic arthroscopy is indicated for those joint conditions that warrant direct examination in order to confirm the presence of clinically suspected disease states that cannot be confirmed by other means of evaluation and where confirmation of the disease will affect the patient's care, or when direct examination will enhance an established diagnosis for purposes of making treatment decisions.[23] Contra-indications include skin infection, possible tumor seeding, and medical or other circumstances unique to the patient. Active ear disease (e.g., otitis media) and compromised neuro-otologic diseases (e.g., Mènière's disease) as well as the presence of major psychological factors in relation to the patient's complaints may be regarded as relative contra-indications.

The surgeon should keep in mind the possibility of inducing iatrogenic damage. Although Holmlund et al. concluded from an experimental study in rabbits that arthroscopic examination was not very invasive,[24] Bjoernland and Rørvik reported irreversible cartilage damage with bone involvement, fibrous tissue formation, and synovial hyperplasia one to three months after arthroscopic inspection with probing of the disc surface in an experimental study in seven goats.[25] Thus, in view of the surgical morbidity of the puncture and surgical intervention in small joints such as the temporomandibular joint, patients should be carefully selected.

Arthroscopic diagnosis and treatment planning in temporomandibular joint degenerative diseases

With the development of diagnostic and surgical arthroscopy, new perspectives have been introduced with regard to temporomandibular joint internal derangement. With successful outcome of arthroscopic surgery aimed at elimination of synovitis and adhesions rather than repositioning of the disc, the significance of disc position has become controversial. Based on the success of arthroscopic lavage of painful and inflamed joints, temporomandibular joint arthrocentesis has become a serious treatment option.

With regard to diagnosis, conventional radiography and computerized tomography adequately detect advanced osteoarthrotic changes. Thus, diagnostic arthroscopy does not seem to be indicated in patients with radiographically obvious temporomandibular joint diseases. However, arthroscopic inspection is useful to assess the presence and severity of synovitis, and detect early degenerative signs such as fibrillation and localized subchondral bone exposure. Diagnostic markers of disease from joint fluid may also appear useful. In future research efforts investigating degenerative diseases without obvious radiographic signs, combined arthroscopic examination and chemical joint fluid analysis may be indicated since the data obtained can be related to the patient's clinical signs and symptoms.

When the arthroscope is applied in diagnosis and treatment planning for temporomandibular joint degenerative diseases, non-surgical diagnostic imaging should be performed first. Diagnostic arthroscopy may be helpful in staging the disease. Specific arthroscopic findings should always be related to the presenting clinical signs and symptoms.

Diagnostic arthroscopy prior to scheduled surgery is indicated in order to relate intra-articular findings to clinical status. Core biopsy studies of the cartilaginous-osseous interface are desirable.

References

1 Ohnishi M. Arthroscopy of the temporomandibular joint (in Japanese). J Jap Stomatol Soc 1975; 42:207

2 Murakami K, Hoshino K. Regional anatomical nomenclature and arthroscopic terminology in human temporomandibular joints. Okajimas Folia Anat Jpn 1982; 58:745

3 Murakami K, Hoshino K. Histological studies on the inner surfaces of the articular cavities of human temporomandibular joints with special reference to the arthroscopic observations. Anat Anz 1985; 160:167

4 Holmlund A, Hellsing G. Arthroscopy of the temporomandibular joint. An autopsy study. Int J Oral Maxillofac Surg 1985; 14:169

5 Holmlund A, Hellsing G, Axelsson S. The temporomandibular joint: a comparison of clinical and arthroscopic findings. J Prosthet Dent 1989; 62:61

6 Sanders B. Arthroscopic surgery of the temporomandibular joint: treatment of internal derangement with persistent closed lock. Oral Surg Oral Med Oral Pathol 1986; 62:361

7 Murakami K, Ono T. Temporomandibular joint arthroscopy by inferolateral approach. Int J Oral Maxillofac Surg 1986; 15:410

8 Kondoh T, Westesson PL. Diagnostic accuracy of temporomandibular joint lower compartment arthroscopy using an ultrathin arthroscope: a postmortem study. J Oral Maxillofac Surg 1991; 49:619

9 Liedberg J, Westesson PL. Diagnostic accuracy of upper compartment arthroscopy of the temporomandibular joint: correlation with postmortem morphology. Oral Surg Oral Med Oral Pathol 1986; 62:618

10 Bibb CA, Pullinger AG, Baldioceda F, Murakami K, Ross J. TMJ comparative imaging: diagnostic efficacy of arthroscopy compared to tomography and arthrography. Oral Surg Oral Med Oral Pathol 1989; 68:352

11 Murakami K, Segami N, Fujimura K, Iizuka T. Correlation between pain and synovitis in patients with internal derangement of the temporomandibular joint. J Oral Maxillofac Surg 1991; 49:1159

12 Merrill RG, Yih WY, Langan M. A histologic evaluation of the accuracy of TMJ diagnostic arthroscopy. Oral Surg Oral Med Oral Pathol 1990; 70:39

13 Holmlund A, Gynther GW, Reinholt FP. Disk derangement and inflammatory changes in the posterior disk attachment of the temporomandibular joint. Oral Surg Oral Med Oral Pathol 1992; 73:9

14 Quinn JH, Bazan NG. Identification of prostaglandin E_2 and leukotrien B_4 in the synovial fluid of painful dysfunctional temporomandibular joints. J Oral Maxillofac Surg 1990; 48:968

15 Holmlund A, Ekblom A, Hansson J, et al. Concentrations of neuropeptides substance P, neurokinin A, calcitonin gene-related peptide, neuropeptide Y and vasoactive intestinal polypeptide in synovial fluid of the human temporomandibular joint. Int J Oral Maxillofac Surg 1991; 20:228

16 Murakami K, Matsuki M, Iizuka T, Ono T. Diagnostic arthroscopy of the TMJ: differential diagnosis in patients with limited jaw opening. J Craniomandibular Pract 1986; 4:117

17 Kaminishi RM, Davis CL. Temporomandibular joint arthroscopic observations of superior space adhesions. Oral Maxillofac Surg Clin North Am 1989; 1:93

18 Murakami K, Segami N, Moriya Y, Iizuka T. Correlation between pain and dysfunction and intra-articular adhesions in patients with internal derangement of the temporomandibular joint. J Oral Maxillofac Surg 1992; 50:705

19 Holmlund A, Hellsing G. Arthroscopy of the temporomandibular joint. Occurrence and location of osteoarthrosis and synovitis in a patient material. Int J Oral Maxillofac Surg 1988; 17:36

20 Quinn JH. Pathogenesis of temporomandibular joint chondromalacia and arthralgia. Oral Maxillofac Surg Clin North Am 1989; 1:47

21 Israel HA, Saed-Nejad F, Ratcliffe A. Early diagnosis of the temporomandibular joint: correlation
    between arthroscopic diagnosis and keratan sulphate levels in the synovial fluid. J Oral Maxillofac
    Surg 1991; 49:708
22 Holmlund A, Gynther G, Reinholt FR. Rheumatoid arthritis and disc derangement of the temporo-
    mandibular joint. A comparative arthroscopic study. Oral Surg Oral Med Oral Pathol 1992; 73:273
23 American Association of Oral and Maxillofacial Surgeons. Position paper on TMJ arthroscopy. J
    Oral Maxillofac Surg 1993; 50 (suppl 7)
24 Holmlund A, Hellsing G, Bang G. Arthroscopy of the rabbit temporomandibular joint. Int J Oral
    Maxillofac Surg 1986; 15:170
25 Bjoenland T, Rørvik M, Haanaes HR, Teige J. Degenerative changes in the temporomandibular
    joint: an experimental study in goats. Int J Oral Maxillofac Surg 1994; 23:41

Surgical procedures: biologic basis and treatment outcome

Management of Temporomandibular
Joint Degenerative Diseases
ed. by B. Stegenga & L.G.M. de Bont
© 1996 Birkhäuser Verlag Basel/Switzerland

Temporomandibular joint arthrocentesis: biologic basis and treatment outcome

Dorrit W. Nitzan

Department of Oral and Maxillofacial Surgery, Faculty of Dental Medicine, The Hebrew University, Hadassah School of Dental Medicine, 91120 Jerusalem, Israel

Summary: Arthrocentesis is an efficient and simple procedure performed under local anesthesia, and has proved to be highly efficacious in releasing severe closed-lock. Biologic mechanisms for the efficacy of arthrocentesis are discussed in this chapter. A treatment protocol, including arthrocentesis in conjuction with occlusal appliance therapy, is suggested.

Introduction

Traditionally, arthrocentesis is a procedure in which the fluid of a joint cavity is aspirated with a needle, through which a required substance is then injected. The procedure is carried out under local anesthesia and under strict sterile conditions, and may be performed repeatedly, if necessary.[1-3] Aspiration of fluid provides important diagnostic information. Aspiration of blood is indicative for hemarthrosis, pus for septic arthritis, and clear fluid is aspirated in non-specific arthritis. Symptomatic relief is dramatic in these disorders or any other acute arthritis.[4] Microscopic analysis provides morphological, microbiological, and biochemical information which may be important for the clinician as well as for research efforts.[5-12]

Temporomandibular joint arthrocentesis was first described systematically by Murakami.[13] The success in relieving closed-lock using his "manipulation technique followed by pumping and hydraulic pressure" was supported by the results achieved by Sanders using arthroscopic lysis and lavage.[14,15] Arthrocentesis as discussed in this chapter is a valuable modification of the traditional method in that two needles rather than one are introduced into the upper joint space. This modification enables joint lavage in addition to fluid aspiration and injection.[16]

For the purpose of this chapter, to elucidate the biologic basis of arthrocentesis, we chose to focus on severe closed-lock, a condition for which arthrocentesis has been found to be highly effective. This method has replaced the usual surgical repositioning and recontouring of the disc, and although it is not geared to change either the shape of the disc or its position, it still has proved highly efficacious in resolving closed-lock for a period of up to 36 months. These unexpected results have opened new avenues of thought regarding the pathogenesis of severe closed-lock and to the development of a working hypothesis that may constitute a possible biologic basis for arthrocentesis.

Arthrocentesis: technique, post-operative care, and clinical experience and outcome

Technique

The patient is seated at a 45-degree angle with the head turned towards the non-affected side to allow an easy approach to the joint. After proper preparation of the target side, the external auditory meatus is blocked with cotton wool soaked in paraffin oil. A line is drawn on the skin from the middle of the tragus to the outer canthus of the eye. The posterior entrance site is located 2 mm below this line at a distance of 10 mm from the center and directly in front of the tragus; the other site is located 10 mm anterior and 10 mm below the line. These sites are marked on the skin and represent the articular fossa and eminence, respectively.[17]

Local anesthesia is applied, avoiding intra-articular injection to permit controlled sampling of synovial fluid. A 19-gauge needle connected to a 1-ml syringe filled with lactated Ringer's solution is inserted into the superior joint compartment at the posterior site. The solution is injected and immediately aspirated, and this procedure is repeated two more times in order to obtain sufficient fluid for diagnostic and research purposes. Next, 2-3 ml of marcaine 0.5% is injected to distend the upper joint space and anesthetize the adjacent tissues. Another 19-gauge needle is inserted into the distended compartment in the area of the articular eminence (anterior entrance site), enabling free flow of Ringer's solution through the superior compartment (figure 1). An infusion bag containing lactated Ringer's solution, placed about 1 meter above the temporo-mandibular joint level, is then connected to one of the needles to allow free flow of about 200 ml of fluid through the joint. On termination of the procedure the needles are removed.

Post-operative care

Post-operative medication consists of anti-inflammatory drugs taken on a regular basis to achieve proper blood levels, and muscle relaxants (e.g., diazepam) taken before bedtime. After two weeks, the dose is gradually reduced according to the patient's needs.

Post-operatively, an occlusal appliance, designed to raise the bite and prevent contact between upper and lower incisors and canines, is inserted. Due to the resulting distalization of the bite force,[18] joint loading is reduced, which contributes to the joint's rehabilitation. The appliance should be left in place around the clock during the first ten post-operative days, then used at night for four additional weeks.

Physical therapy exercises are performed to stretch and strengthen the muscles surrounding the temporomandibular joint. Maximal opening, latero-trusive, and protrusive movements are performed unresisted, resisted, and

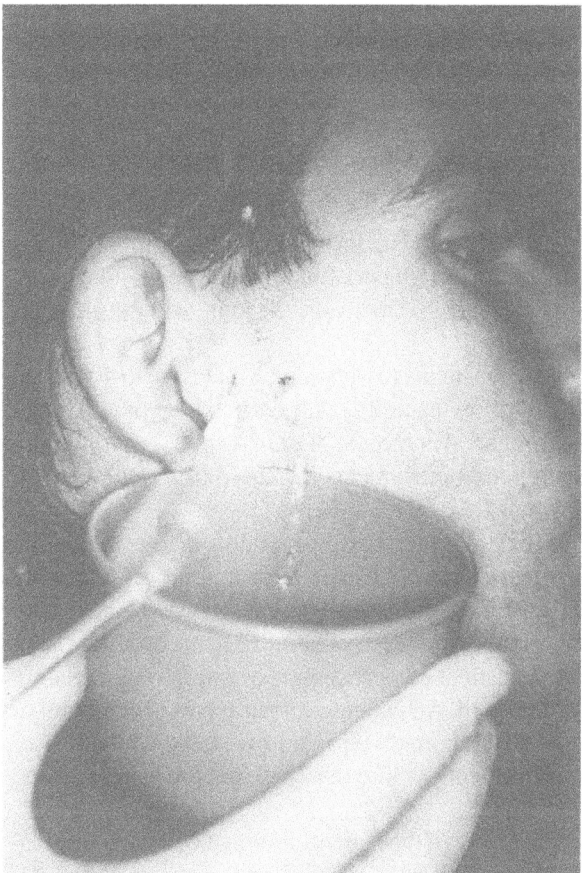

Figure 1.
Two needles inserted at two sites of entrance (fossa and eminence regions) allowing free flow of the injected fluid.

using passive stretch after reaching the maximal active range of movement. Each exercise is repeated ten times, and each series of exercises is performed six times a day during the first two weeks after treatment, after which the program is adjusted individually.

In order to maintain the improvement achieved during the arthrocentesis procedure, strict adherence to the post-operative protocol is imperative.

Clinical experience and outcome

Patient evaluation is based on data obtained during careful anamnesis and clinical examination, entered on a standardized questionnaire by the examiner. In addition, patient self-assessment using a facial diagram and visual analog scales greatly enhances patient evaluation.[19]

Criteria for the diagnosis 'severe closed-lock' include persistent, sudden,

and disabling, but not necessarily painful, restriction of maximal mouth opening to less than 30 mm. To verify that the restriction originates within the joint,
a restricted laterotrusive movement of the jaw towards the unaffected side and
a jaw deviation towards the affected side on opening and protrusive movement
must be present. In addition, joint pain or pressure is elicited by forceful passive
stretch after maximal active opening.

Reports on the effectivity of arthrocentesis in the treatment of severe
closed-lock have been published.[13,16,20] The techniques used in these studies
are based on similar principles, i.e., introducing fluid into the upper joint space
to increase the intra-articular pressure and to lavage the joint, without attempt-
ing to change disc shape or position.

The author has followed up 39 patients (31 females, 8 males) with 40 locked
joints for almost 40 months.[17] Following arthrocentesis, maximal mouth opening increased significantly from an average of 23.1 mm (s.d. 5.2 mm) to 44.3
mm (s.d. 5.0 mm), and contralateral movements increased from 4.8 mm (s.d.
2.4 mm) to 8.2 mm (s.d. 1.9 mm).

In addition to these objective improvements, we found a marked reduction
in pain rate (85%) and dysfunction rate (72%) as measured on visual analog
scales. Dysfunction following treatment, when present, was associated with
reappearance of joint clicking rather than restricted movement capacity. Using
another visual analog scale, the patient's improvement or deterioration relating
to pain and dysfunction was assessed. All patients but one reported an improvement. Twenty-two patients (55%) reported 100% improvement, while 90% of
the patients reported an improvement of more than 75% in both pain level and
dysfunction rate.

It should be emphasized that none of the patients returned with their original
problem; with increasing follow-up time, a marked increase in the patients'
mouth opening and contralateral movement capacity was observed, associated
with a significant improvement in pain and dysfunction rates. Patients older
than 40 years achieved the same results as did younger patients, though at a
slower pace.

Twelve joints (30%) did not click either before the locking occurred or
following its release by arthrocentesis. The other joints clicked before they
locked. In 25 of these 28 joints (89%) clicking had disappeared following
arthrocentesis, while these 25 patients showed a mean maximal mouth opening
of 44.7 mm (s.d. 5.4 mm, range 38-58 mm). These findings do not support the
widely accepted concept of closed-lock being a stage in the natural history of
temporomandibular joint internal derangements.

The percentage of success of arthrocentesis is similar to that reported for
arthroscopic lysis and lavage.[4] It is reasonable to assume that a major part of
the success of surgical arthroscopy in severe closed-lock can be attributed to
the lavage rather than to surgical instrumentation. The benefit of viewing the
surgical field probably does not contribute to the outcome to any appreciable
extent. Moreover, surgical arthroscopy seems to be associated with a certain
amount of scar formation, since the mean maximal mouth opening at follow-up

is less than that immediately following treatment.[4] The data confirm that lavage of the upper joint compartment performed under local anesthesia provides a simple and inexpensive relief of severe closed-lock.

Discussion

Arthrocentesis is capable of releasing severe closed-lock without changing either the shape of the disc or its position.[16,19-24] Since much remains to be investigated, we are forced to construct a working hypothesis of the biologic basis of arthrocentesis in closed-lock.

Traditionally, closed-lock is considered a consequence of a non-reducing deformed disc acting as an obstacle to the sliding condylar head.[25-30] As a consequence, non-surgical or, when this fails, surgical disc repositioning is considered necessary in order to re-establish normal maximal mouth opening.[31-33] This concept was first challenged in 1991, based on findings that were not compatible with a dislocated disc obstructing condylar movement.[28] These findings demonstrate that there is a group of patients with a mouth-opening restriction that is too extreme to be explained simply by a non-reducing deformed disc. It has been argued that the disc is totally prevented from sliding in cases with extreme restriction of movement. Recent studies have revealed that severe closed-lock may arise in temporomandibular joints with normally shaped discs,[28] and even in joints with non-displaced discs without a history of clicking prior to locking.[16,17] The remarkably high success rate in releasing a severe closed-lock without any relapse by arthroscopic lavage and lysis,[14,15,19,34,35] pressure injections,[13,20] and arthrocentesis[16,17] places the original concept in a doubtful light, especially after it has been shown by arthrography and magnetic resonance imaging studies that the position of the disc remains unaffected following these procedures.[20-23,28]

Increased friction and low viscosity of the synovial fluid have been proposed as etiological factors in joints with closed-lock. It has been shown, however, that no matter by what proportion friction is increased, it will always remain insufficient to withstand muscle forces.[36] It also seems unlikely that a decrease in synovial fluid viscosity is associated with a closed-lock, since during arthrocentesis saline, which has a low viscosity, does not only disrupt joint lubrication but also quite easily resolves a locked joint.

Sanders was the first propose a 'suction-cup effect' as interference with normal disc sliding.[15] His assumption was supported by the relatively high negative pressures measured in the upper compartment of temporomandibular joints with severe closed-lock.[36] The suction-cup effect in our opinion represents a stage in the sequence of events leading to impeded joint movement. It may be the consequence of a condition which transmits increased forces across the joint (e.g., parafunctions, such as clenching).[18] We have measured a mean intra-articular pressure in temporomandibular joints with various disorders of 63.4 mm Hg (s.d. 51.6 mm Hg, range 8-220 mm Hg).[18] Assuming a direct relationship of intra-articular pressure with joint loading, this can be sufficient to press and tightly adapt the biconcave disc against the posterior slope of the articular eminence (figure 2A and 2B). On load removal the disc will resume its original shape (figure 2C), and in case of sudden severe closed-lock the central portion of the disc separates from the eminence leaving the rims adapted to the surface increasing the negative pressure within the closed space between disc and eminence slope. It is assumed that condylar rotation in the lower joint compartment is retained in case of a sudden severe closed-lock, while any attempt of the inferior head of the lateral pterygoid muscle to elicit condylar

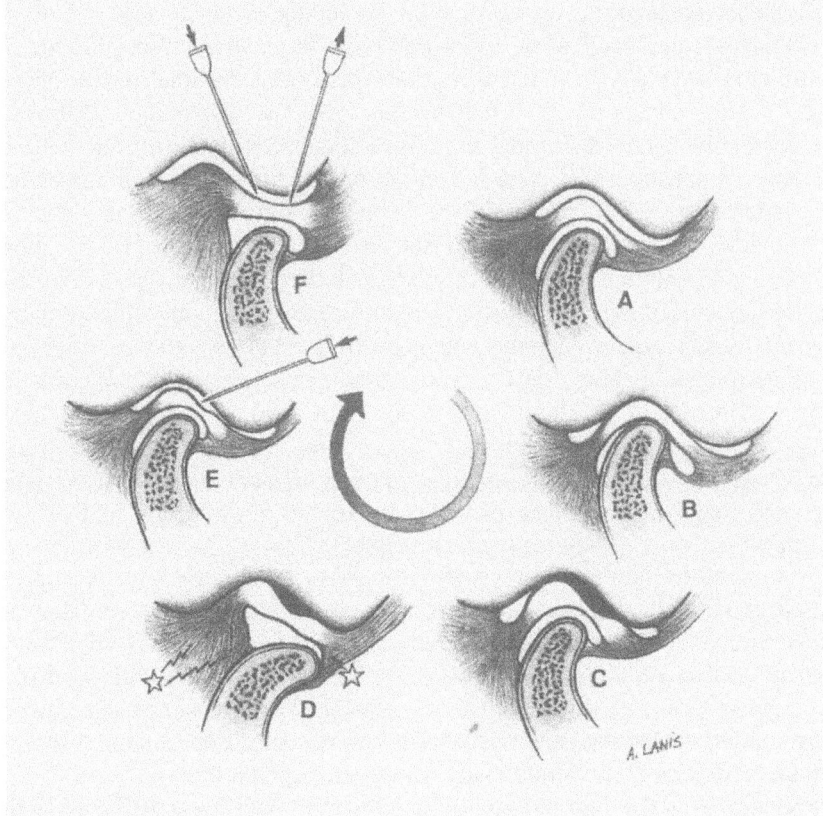

Figure 2.
Proposed sequence of events in the creation and release of a vacuum between disc and eminence (suction-cup effect).
A. Normal temporomandibular joint, showing condyle, disc, retrodiscal tissue, eminence, and fossa.
B. Disc pressed flat against the slope of the eminence.
C. Vacuum effect (dark area).
D. Lateral pterygoid muscle pull (*) induces stretching of capsule, giving rise to pain and reflex inhibition of lateral pterygoid activity.
E. Release of vacuum by insertion of needle between disc and eminence.
F. Reformation of upper joint space allowing free sliding movements following arthrocentesis.

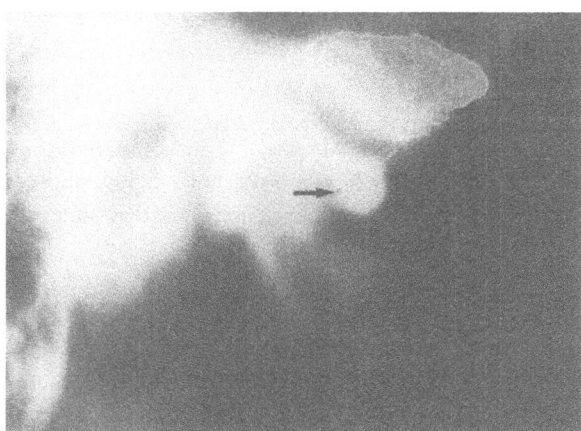

Figure 3.
Arthrogram of a temporo-
mandibular joint with
internal derangement with
deformation (arrow) and
overstretched appearance of
inferior compartment.

sliding is resisted by the firmly anchored disc. As a result, the highly innervated non-elastic lower stratum of the retrodiscal tissue and the capsule are stretched. This causes pain, thus eliciting a reflex that prevents the muscle from exerting sufficient force to overcome the resistance caused by the vacuum phenomenon (figure 2D). As long as the disc is anchored, any attempt of the patient to open the mouth is associated with gradual stretching of the disc attachments to the condylar head, which disrupts the tight relationship between disc and condyle resulting in an undesirable structural change of the lower compartment, as can be arthrographically shown (figure 3). These changes probably cause pain and dysfunction which remains following arthrocentesis, especially in patients with long-standing untreated severe closed-lock. We therefore recommend avoiding delay in performing arthrocentesis and discourage physiotherapy prior to arthrocentesis.

The negative pressure in the upper joint compartment has been shown to be eliminated after introducing a needle (figure 2E).[36] Sliding is reinstituted only after lavage is performed (figure 2F). Thus, besides the negative pressure, other factors keep the disc and eminence attached to one another. These unknown factors constitute the biologic basis for arthrocentesis. We constructed a working hypothesis based on the clinical presentation of closed-lock, its predisposing factors, and its response to arthrocentesis, as well as on the relevant literature regarding other synovial joints.

The harmful potential of loading (e.g., clenching) is well established.[37] In order to verify the relationship between clenching and closed-lock, intra-articular pressure was measured during clenching, rest, and maximal mouth opening.[18] Intra-articular pressure during clenching was high enough (63.4 mm Hg, s.d. 51.6 mm Hg) to press the condyle firmly against the eminence. Moreover, this pressure may cause temporary hypoxia, taking into account that the hydrostatic pressure in normal capillaries is about 30 mm Hg, increasing to 60 mm Hg in inflamed tissue. At rest, the intra-articular pressure is released and reperfusion occurs. During maximal mouth opening the intra-articular pressure reduces to negative levels (–54.0 mm Hg, s.d. 35.5 mm Hg), inducing further perfusion. The biochemistry of this hypoxic-re-oxygenation cycle is now well known, involving the production of insulting oxygen-derived free radicals which were shown in inflamed joints during exercise.[38-40] Inflammation may activate a variety of biochemical changes which are presently being studied, and which we consider major contributors to the persistence of the disc adhering to the articular eminence.

Arthrocentesis abolishes the negative pressure, relieves the adhered disc, and probably also drains inflammatory and pain mediators from the joint, thus bringing about recovery of normal joint function.[18] An important aspect is that the synovial fluid is eliminated during arthrocentesis; nevertheless, free condyle-disc sliding is not disrupted and even improves. What factors are responsible for joint lubrication and the precise role of the synovial fluid remain topics for further study.

Although arthrocentesis provides a symptomatic solution for severe closed-lock, it does not eliminate its underlying cause(s). Control of detrimental forces from clenching is warranted as an adjunct to arthrocentesis. An occlusal appliance, specifically designed to diminish joint loading, reduces the pressure generated in the upper joint compartment during clenching by 81% (figure 4A and 4B). The appliance most probably contributes to preventing a restart of the

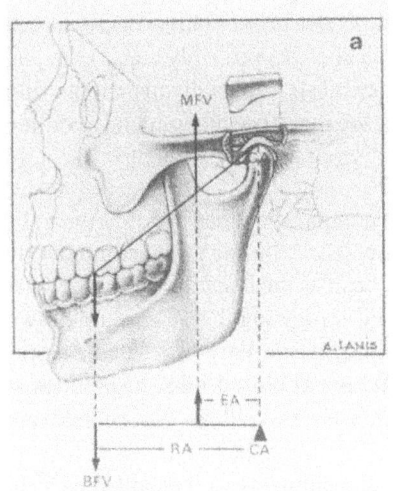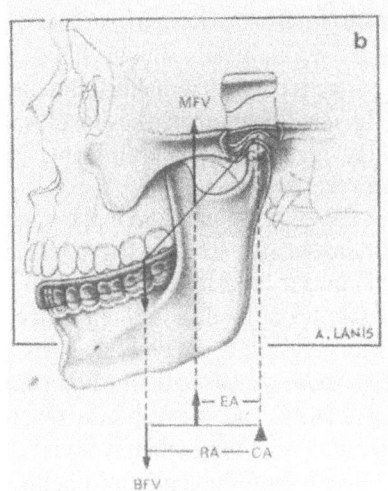

Figure 4.
Mandible in clenched position.
A. Without occlusal appliance.
B. With occlusal appliance: contact between upper and lower front teeth is prevented, thereby distalizing bite force vector (BFV) and shortening of the resistance arm (RA) relative to unchanged effort arm (EA) with resultant decreased force directed toward condylar axis (CA), i.e. temporomandibular joint loading.

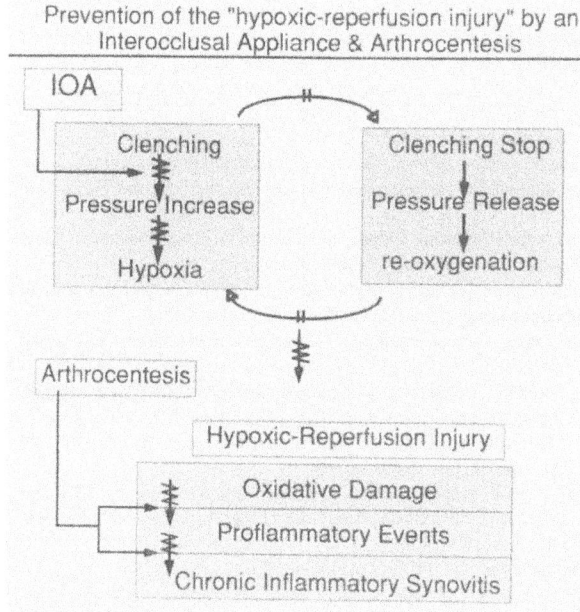

Figure 5.
Prevention of 'hypoxic-reperfusion injury' by arthrocentesis and an occlusal appliance.

hypoxic-reperfusion cycle, thus preserving the results obtained during arthrocentesis and preventing recurrence of inflammation or closed-lock (figure 5).

References

1 Brown PW. Arthrocentesis for diagnosis and therapy. Surg Clin North Am 1969; 49:1269
2 Geigerman JM, Dawson WJ. Diagnostic arthrocentesis: indications and method. Postgrad Med 1979; 66:141
3 Samuelson CO Jr, Cannon GW, Ward JR. Arthrocentesis. J Fam Pract 1985; 20:179
4 Nitzan DW. Arthrocentesis for the management of severe closed lock. Oral Maxillofac Surg Clin North Am 1994; 6:245
5 Rossomando EF, White LB, Hadjimichael J, et al. Immunomagnetic separation of tumor necrosis factor alpha. I. Batch procedure for human temporomandibular fluid. J Chromoatogr 1992; 583:11
6 Appelgren A, Appelgren B, Eriksson S, et al. Neuropeptides in temporomandibular joints with rheumatoid arthritis: a clinical study. Scand J Dent Res 1991; 99:519
7 Holmlund A, Ekblom A, Hansson P, et al. Concentration of neuropeptides substance P, neurokinin A, calcitonin related peptide, neuropeptide Y and vasoactive intestinal polypeptide in synovial fluid of the human temporomandibular joint. A correlation with symptoms, signs and arthroscopic findings. Int J Oral Maxillofac Surg 1991; 20:228
8 Israel HA, Saed-Nejad F, Ratcliffe A. Early diagnosis of osteoarthrosis of the temporomandibular joint: correlation between arthroscopic diagnosis and keratan sulphate levels in the synovial fluid. J Oral Maxillofac Surg 1991; 49:708
9 Israel HA. Synovial fluid analysis. Oral Maxillofac Surg Clin North Am 1989; 1:85
10 Smith AJ, Basu MK, Speculand B, et al. Synovial fluid glycosaminoglycan (acid mucopolysaccharide) analysis in assessment of temporomandibular joint dysfunction. A pilot study. Br J Oral Maxillofac Surg 1989; 27:853

11 Ratcliffe A, Doherty M, Maini RN. Increased concentrations of proteoglycan components in the synovial fluid of patients with acute but not chronic joint disease. Ann Rheum Dis 1988; 47:826

12 Kopp S, Wenneberg B, Clemensson E. Clinical, microscopical and biochemical investigation of synovial fluid from temporomandibular joints. Scand J Dent Res 1983; 91:33

13 Murakami KI, Matsuki M, Iizuka T, et al. Recapturing the persistent anterior displaced disk by mandibular manipulation after pumping and hydraulic pressure to the upper joint cavity of the temporomandibular joint. J Craniomandibular Pract 1987; 5:18

14 Sanders B, Buoncristiani R. Diagnostic and surgical arthroscopy of the temporomandibular joint: clinical experience with 137 procedures over a 2-year period. J Craniomandib Disord Facial Oral Pain 1987; 1:202

15 Sanders N. Arthroscopic surgery of the temporomandibular joint: treatment of internal derangement with persistent closed-lock. Oral Surg Oral Med Oral Pathol 1986; 62:361

16 Nitzan DW, Dolwick MF, Martinet GA. Temporomandibular joint arthrocentesis: a simplified treatment for severe limited mouth opening. J Oral Maxillofac Surg 1991; 48:1163

17 McCain JP. Arthroscopy of the human temporomandibular joint. J. Oral Maxillofac Surg 1988; 46:648

18 Nitzan DW. Intra-articular pressures in the functioning human temporomandibular joint and their alteration with uniformly raised mandibular occlusal plane. J Oral Maxillofac Surg 1994; 52:671

19 Nitzan DW, Dolwick MF, Heft MW. Arthroscopic lavage and lysis of the temporomandibular joint: a change in perspective. J Oral Maxillofac Surg 1990; 48:796

20 Segami N, Murakami KI, Iizuka T. Arthrographic evaluation of disk position following mandibular manipulation technique for internal derangement with closed lock of the temporomandibular joint. J Craniomandib Disord Facial Oral Pain 1990; 4:99

21 Bronstein SL. Postsurgical TMJ arthrography. J Craniomandibular Pract 1984; 2:165

22 Gabler MJ, Greene CS, Palacios E. Effect of arthroscopic temporomandibular joint surgery on articular disk position. J Craniomandib Disord Facial Oral Pain 1989; 3:191

23 Mongomery MT, Van Sickels JE, Harms SE, et al. Arthroscopic TMJ surgery: effects on signs, symptoms, and disc position. J Oral Maxillofac Surg 1989; 47:1263

24 Moses JJ, Sartoris D, Glass R. The effect of arthroscopic surgical lysis and lavage of the superior joint space on TMJ disc position and mobility. J Oral Maxillofac Surg 1989; 47:674

25 Dolwick MF, Katzberg RW. Helms CA. Internal derangement of the temporomandibular joint. Fact or fiction? J Prosthet Dent 1983; 49:415

26 Farrar WB. Characteristic of the condylar path in internal derangement of the TMJ. J Prosthet Dent 1978; 39:319

27 Ireland WE. The problem of "the clicking jaw". Proc R Soc Med 1951; 44;363

28 Nitzan DW, Dolwick MF. An alternative explanation for the genesis of closed-lock symptoms in the internal derangement process. J Oral Maxillofac Surg 1991; 49:810

29 Westesson PL, Bronstein SL, Liedberg J. Internal derangement of the temporomandibular joint. Morphologic description with correlation to joint function. Oral Surg Oral Med Oral Pathol 1985; 59:323

30 Wilkes CH. Internal derangement of the temporomandibular joint. Archs Otolaryng Head Neck Surg 1989; 115;469

31 Dolwick MF, Sanders B. TMJ internal derangement & arthrosis. Surgical atlas. St Louis: Mosby, 1985

32 Laskin DM. Surgery of the temporomandibular joint. In: Temporomandibular joint problems. Biologic diagnosis and treatment. Solberg WK, Clark GT (eds). Chicago: Quintessence, 1980; 111

33 McCarty WL, Farrar WB. Surgery for internal derangement of the temporomandibular joint. J Prosthet Dent 1979; 42:191

34 Davis CL, Kaminishi RM, Marshall MW. Arthroscopic surgery for treatment of closed lock. J Oral Maxillofac Surg 1991; 49:704

35 Indresano AT. Arthroscopic surgery of the temporomandibular joint: report of 64 patients with long-term follow-up. J Oral Maxillofac Surg 1989; 47:439

36 Nitzan DW, Mahler Y, Simkin A. Intra-articular pressure measurements in patients with suddenly developing, severely limited mouth opening. J Oral Maxillofac Surg 1992; 50:1038

37 Rugh JD, Ohrbach R. Occlusal parafunction. In: Textbook of occlusion. Mohl ND, Zarb GA, Carlsson GE, Rugh JD (eds). Chicago: Quintessence, 1988; 81

38 Blake DR, Merry P. Unsworth F. Hypoxia-reperfusion injury in the inflamed human joint. Lancet 1989; 111:289

39 Woodruff T, Blak DR, Freeman F, Andrews PS. Is chronic synovitis an example of reperfusion injury? Ann Rheum Dis 1986; 45:608
40 Merry P, Williams R, Cox N, et al. Comparative study of intra-articular pressure dynamics in joints with acute traumatic and chronic inflammatory effusion. Potential implications for hypoxic reperfusion injury. Ann Rheum Dis 1991; 50:917

Management of Temporomandibular
Joint Degenerative Diseases
ed. by B. Stegenga & L.G.M. de Bont
© 1996 Birkhäuser Verlag Basel/Switzerland

Biologic basis and outcome of arthroscopic lysis and lavage of the temporomandibular joint

Robert D. Schwartz

Department of Oral and Maxillofacial Surgery, University of Illinois and Northwestern University, Chicago, Illinois 60602, USA

Summary: In clinical and imaging studies, an increase in range of motion, improvement of joint function, and reduction of pain was observed after lysis of adhesions and lavage of the superior temporomandibular joint compartment. The successful surgical outcome can be explained by the effects of washing out mediators of pain and inflammation, improved mobility, and adaptive mechanisms rather than restoration of disc position.

Introduction

Prior to the introduction of arthroscopy of the temporomandibular joint those patients who were diagnosed with internal derangement and/or osteoarthrosis who fulfilled the criteria for surgical intervention would undergo a variety of procedures primarily based on the preference and experience of the surgeon. The procedures performed consisted of disc repair, discectomy with temporary or permanent alloplastic replacement, discectomy with autogenous replacement, discectomy with no replacement, eminectomy, and condylar shave. The surgical outcome of a significant number of these patients was disappointing due to the fact that the sequelae of these procedures frequently exhibited progressive degeneration of the operated joint. Many of these patients experienced multiple procedures and ultimately went on to total joint replacement. In addition, skeletal jaw deformities developed secondary to loss of condylar mass.

Arthroscopy of the temporomandibular joint was introduced in the 1980s by Ohnishi,[1] Kino,[2] Murakami et al.,[3] and Holmlund and Hellsing.[4] From preliminary investigations of the therapeutic benefits, arthroscopy appeared to be a less invasive technique that has the potential of successful surgical outcome with minimal sequelae.

The primary procedure performed was lysis and lavage of the superior joint compartment with or without intra-capsular injection of a steroid. Studies comparing the pre- and post-operative imaging status demonstrated very little improvement of disc position.[5-9] However, an increase in range of motion, improvement of joint function, and reduction of pain was significantly observed from this basic procedure. It became clear that the successful surgical outcome may not be predicated on the restoration of disc position. Other factors may play a more important role in improving range of motion and joint function, and reducing pain.

Significant progress has been made in understanding the pathophysiology of temporomandibular disorders. When treating patients with internal derangements, this particular finding by virtue of its definition may be inadequate because of the many other concomitant findings associated with internal derangements, such as synovitis, adherence of discal tissue and its attachments to the articular cartilage of the temporal bone, fibrous connective tissue adhesions, chondromalacia, osteoarthrosis, haemarthrosis, capsular fibrosis, and dystrophic calcifications.

Pathophysiologic processes in temporomandibular joint degenerative diseases

The basic structures of synovial joints include articular cartilage, disc, synovium, capsule, and subchondral bone. The articulating structures require a thin layer of healthy synovial fluid for an optimal functional relationship allowing for low-friction load-bearing.[10] Effective joint lubrication is accomplished through a complex biomechanical mechanism and, although not fully understood, is imperative for normal function.[11,12] The functional demands placed on synovial joints elicit biochemical, biomechanical and biosynthetic adaptive mechanisms (remodeling and reparative processes) from these structures.

Connective tissue cells in both condensed and loose tissues are embedded in an abundant extracellular matrix composed of collagen, proteoglycans, elastin, fibronectin, and other proteins. The majority of connective tissues have a great regenerative capacity, displaying remarkable cellular proliferation and biosynthetic activity, particularly in response to injury. Under normal conditions a relatively active turnover exists, with continuous degradation and replacement of macromolecular components. When the physiologic limits of adaptive capacity (repair and remodeling) of the joint structures are exceeded, a degradation process prevails. This process consists of complex interactions between biomechanical, biochemical, inflammatory, immunologic, and metabolic reactions that can lead to dysfunctional and disease states. In diffuse connective tissue diseases, critical events take place, not only in the synovium but also in the interstitial tissue throughout the body. The interaction between the primary cellular and macromolecular components of the connective tissue (fibroblasts and their relatives, extracellular proteins, and ground substance) and inflammatory cells (monocytes, lymphocytes, mast cells, and polymorphonuclear leucocytes) and their products is probably crucial to the pathogenesis and outcome of many rheumatic diseases.[13,14] Degradative enzymes located in the chondrocytes of the articular cartilage and the cells of the synovial membrane are capable of breaking down proteoglycans. Cytokines from the synovial lining activate the chondrocytes to produce collagenase and a neutral metalloprotease, which perpetuates the degradation process of the articular cartilage.[15-17]

These degradative mechanisms can alter and affect the integrity of the articular cartilage (chondromalacia), the cellular response of the synovium (nutritional and lubrication deficiency, inflammation, activation of degradative enzymes, and fibrosis), the disc (position, mobility, morphology, and histopathology), the capsule (fibrosis and contracture), and the subchondral bone (microfractures, osteophyte formation, subchondral cysts, and eburnation), as seen in osteoarthrosis.

Several physiologic processes contribute to the normal dynamics of the temporomandibular joint. When these processes are interfaced with systemic disease or localized pathology and dysfunction, pathophysiologic processes become involved, including nutritional deprivation of articular cartilage and disc, impairment of joint lubrication, inflammation, proliferation of fibrous connective tissue adhesions, the activation and synthesis of degradative enzymes, and destruction of local tissues by free oxygen radicals known as ischemia-reperfusion injury.[18-20]

The effects of the inflammatory process on synovial joints as a result of the pathophysiologic processes described would be best summarized by

- alteration of synovial fluid viscosity leading to impairment of lubrication and nutrition to the articular cartilage and disc
- activation of degradative enzymes which have deleterious effects on synovium and articular cartilage
- fibrosis of the synovial membrane in the form of adhesions
- reactive and proliferative forms of synovitis.[21]

The etiopathogenesis of osteoarthrosis takes on several possible theories:[22,23]

- abrasion and breakdown of the surface of the articular cartilage due to increased frictional wear and tear secondary to repetitive overloading resulting in decreased collagen network stiffness which leads to increased hydration of the proteoglycan-water gel.
- inability of cartilage cells to produce adequate matrix components.
- microfractures of the subchondral bone secondary to stiffening and overloading of the joint with subsequent cartilaginous breakdown and a synovial inflammatory response.[23,24]
- disturbance of articular cartilage homeostasis by biochemical activity in the form of cytokine activity, growth factors, degradative enzymes, mediators for pain and inflammation, and the effects of inflammation on synovial fluid.[25-27]

It appears logical that investigations need to be directed toward developing an appreciation of those factors that interfere with joint lubrication and the effects of these factors on joint mobility, pain and function, and to verify whether the temporomandibular joint and its associated musculoskeletal components obey the same biological laws that other synovial articulation obey, as proposed by

Stegenga, de Bont and Boering.[28] Recently several studies have evolved from the oral and maxillofacial surgery literature regarding biochemical activities of the temporomandibular joint.[29-32] Such studies need to be encouraged and continued to ascertain scientific information relative to the pathophysiology of temporomandibular arthropathies.

Biologic basis for arthroscopic lysis and lavage

The biologic basis for arthroscopic lysis and lavage appears to be based on several factors.

Joint lubrication,[11,12] which is imperative for normal joint function, becomes impaired secondary to an inflammatory process. Pathological synovial fluids exhibit diminished viscosity due to a decreased hyaluronate concentration. Under these conditions the functional integrity of the synovial lining and articular surfaces are vulnerable to increased frictional wear and abrasion as they slide by each other. The reduction of synovial fluid viscosity leads to irritation of the synovial lining, which perpetuates the inflammatory process. Leakage of proteoglycans into the joint space as a result of late stage chondromalacia also is an irritation to the synovial lining. Lavaging the pathological synovial fluid provides an environment for the synthesis of healthy synovial fluid. Washing out the mediators of pain and inflammation can also create an environment for anabolic repair.

The separation of the superior surface of the disc and its attachments that are adherent to the temporal articulating surface (lysis) eliminates the resistance the condyle meets during translation. Mechanical resistance to condylar translation appears to be secondary to alterations of synovial fluid viscosity and/or connective tissue adhesions that are impairing the mobility of the disc and its attachments and secondarily interfering with condylar mobility (figure 1).[9,33,34]

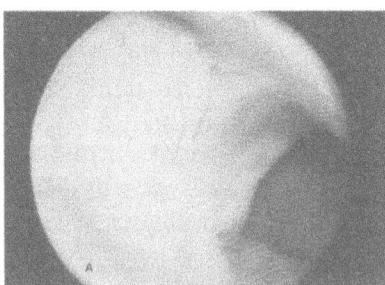 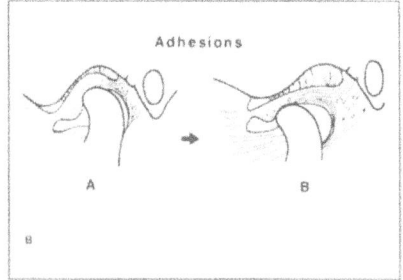

Figure 1.
Adhesions – the result of an inflammatory process.
A. Fibrous adhesion in the anterior recess of the upper joint space.
B. Schematic representation of the influence adhesions have on condylar mobility. Note the resistance the condyle meets upon opening from the immobilized disc and its attachments which is adherent to the glenoid fossa and posterior slope of the eminence (Courtesy of Dr. Bruce Sanders).

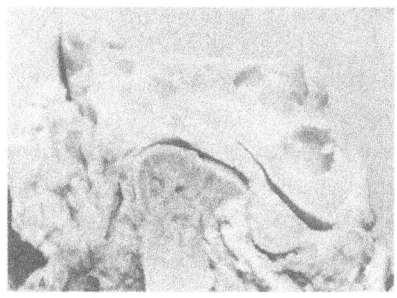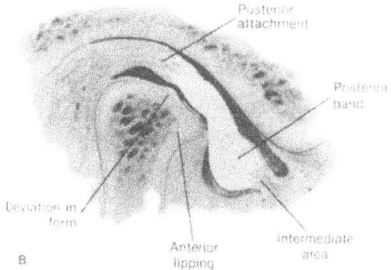

Figure 2.
Functional remodeling and adaptation of an osteoarthrotic temporomandibular joint.
A. Cadaveric specimen of an osteoarthrotic joint demonstrating an intact cortex associated with a functionally remodeled condyle, glenoid fossa, and adapted retrodiscal tissue.
B. Schematic representation (Courtesy of Dr. M. Franklin Dolwick).

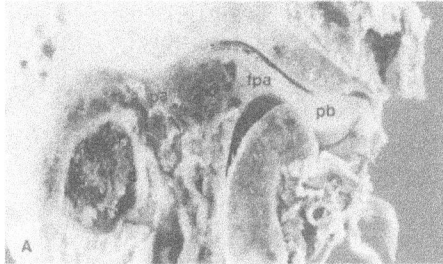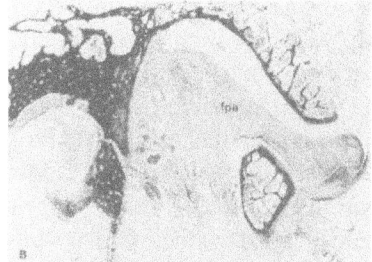

Figure 3.
A. Adaptation of retrodiscal tissue (fpa) of cadaveric specimen with internal derangement of right temporomandibular joint. Note that the posterior band (pb) has undergone morphologic deformation and is located anterior to the condyle.
B. Histologic section of A demonstrating fibrosis of the retrodiscal tissue (fpa), illustrating adaptation potential of retrodiscal tissue (Courtesy of Dr. M. Franklin Dolwick).

The potential of the retrodiscal tissue to adapt to 'disc-like' tissue secondary to metaplastic changes provide an environment for the joint to be loaded on tissue that can safely withstand functional loading (figure 2).[35,36] In certain patient populations the disc may not need to be in a normal relationship for a patient to have successful surgical outcome with an increased range of motion, reduction of pain, and normal functional loading (figure 3).

Treatment outcome of arthroscopic lysis and lavage

Most of the clinical studies on lysis and lavage are largely descriptive methodologic articles or retrospective case reviews compiled by surgeons themselves. Such case reviews provide valuable initial data about a new procedure, but are subject to bias and may not yield a careful evaluation of the procedure. No truly controlled blind studies have been published.

Sanders and Buoncristiani reported the outcome of 340 arthroscopies (34 diagnostic only, 306 therapeutic as well) in 213 patients (198 females, 15 males, mean age 30 years) with symptoms of preauricular pain and mandibular hypomobility secondary to internal derangement with persistent closed-lock or osteoarthrosis with adhesive capsulitis for which non-surgical therapy has been unsuccessful.[37] Of the 221 joints with closed lock, 213 (96.4%) had a successful result, characterized by increase in mandibular opening, mobility, function, and decreased pain and disability. Seventy-nine of the 85 joints with osteoarthrosis were successful (92.9%). In total, 14 of 306 joints that underwent arthroscopic lysis and lavage failed (4.5%). The results of arthroscopic lysis and lavage in the treatment of 26 painful joints after previous arthrotomy (excluding implants) were rated as poor in only one case in Sanders' series.

Moses and Poker conducted a study on 237 patients with a non-reducing disc displacement (confirmed with arthrography or magnetic resonance imaging) who underwent lysis and lavage.[38] Ninety-seven percent of the patients that were studied felt the surgery was a success, and 82% said they would have the surgery again.

White reported a retrospective analysis of 100 consecutive surgical arthroscopies.[39] The mean post-operative increase in maximal interincisal opening was 38.4%. A 7.5% failure rate was noted by objective criteria and 85.7% of the patients rated their post-operative pain and function greatly or moderately improved. All the respondents stated that they would have the arthroscopic surgery again if needed.

Montgomery et al. reported excellent clinical results with arthroscopic lysis and lavage, even though there was not a significant reduction of the displaced disc.[7] Indresano reported the outcome of 100 temporomandibular joint arthroscopies.[40] A gain in maximal interincisal opening of 50%, and a reduction of pain greater than 70% or greater was considered successful. In addition, any case requiring additional surgery within a two-year period was considered a failure. An overall success rate of 73% was obtained for all surgical arthroscopic procedures. Persistent closed-lock was found to be the most predictable successful condition treated with a therapeutic success of 83%. Those patients who underwent arthroscopic lysis and lavage for painful clicking joints; only 50% of those fulfilled a satisfactory result. Israel and Roser reported similar findings with a relief of symptoms and increased range of motion in a study of 24 patients who underwent arthroscopic lysis and lavage (28 joints).[41] Nitzan and Dolwick presented a study of 30 patients (28 joints) who underwent lysis and lavage, and reported an overall success rate of 70%.[42]

Perrott reported a prospective evaluation of the effectiveness of temporomandibular joint arthroscopy.[43] At early (10-30 days), intermediate (1-6 months), and late (more than 6 months) follow-up increase in maximal opening was statistically significant. Noise did not return in the majority of patients. Disc position, evaluated by magnetic resonance imaging in 29 joints, did not appear to change in 25 joints. Clark and Liu performed a prospective study of long-term outcome (two years) for 18 patients, which was neither a controlled nor randomized trial.[44] The mean pain score at the final assessment had decreased by 57%. Jaw function showed an average improvement of 67%, and maximal active opening ability showed a 13 mm increase. Davis et al. evaluated 51 consecutive cases (80 joints) treated for restriction of mandibular opening due to closed-lock.[45] The results showed an immediate improvement after arthroscopic lysis and lavage, followed by more gradual improvement during the next six months with a plateau improvement thereafter. Moore conducted a prospective longitudinal study in 63 consecutive patients (mean age 35.7 years, 92% female), admitted to the study for three years.[46] Arthroscopic lysis and lavage was performed in 120 temporomandibular joints. Mandibular range of motion improved rapidly following arthroscopic surgery, stabilizing at about 8-10 weeks post-operatively. Pain showed the greatest improvement within the first four weeks, improved more gradually until six months, then stabilizing. Subjective dysfunction improved less rapidly. Of the patients accepted in the study protocol, 87% had successful result at one year. This percentage remained successful at two years after surgery, and no additional failures were seen thereafter.

A retrospective study by Zeitler and Porter not only demonstrated the effectiveness of arthroscopic lysis and lavage, but also demonstrated the effectiveness in a comparable procedure for arthrotomy and disc repositioning.[47] The results revealed that 79% of the arthroscopy patients and 76% of the arthrotomy patients were treated successfully. This small difference was not statistically significant. The results indicate that arthroscopic surgery is an alternative to arthrotomy for certain conditions of the temporomandibular joint. Arthroscopic surgery appears to be effective in eliminating pain and restoring mandibular function when non-surgical therapy has failed, particularly in patients exhibiting non-reducing anterior disc displacement. Aside from a pre-operative diagnosis of permanent disc displacement, another factor that may influence the therapeutic success of a procedure is the pre-operative duration of symptoms. A shorter pre-operative duration of symptoms was found to result in a more favorable therapeutic outcome for arthrotomy patients. Early surgical intervention is more likely to result in a successful therapeutic outcome for this procedure.

Stegenga conducted a study on the short-term outcome of arthroscopic surgery in a randomized controlled clinical trial.[48] Inclusion and exclusion criteria were specifically defined, and 28 subjects were randomly assigned to the therapeutic groups (arthroscopic surgery, non-surgical treatment). One of the important results of this study is that the treatment responses appeared to be independent of the treatment type, which suggests that all forms of therapy are more or less capable of reducing symptoms. The results of this study, although based on a small sample, support the importance of and the need for controlled studies.

Conclusion

Data from retrospective and prospective studies support the conclusion that arthroscopic lysis and lavage can be a very effective procedure for the improvement of range of motion, joint function, and a decrease in arthralgia in a significant number of patients with painful hypomobility and temporomandibular joint degenerative disease. One of the dilemmas is why a significant number of patients have the adaptive capacity to heal and function uneventfully and then there are those who undergo progressive degeneration of their joints, even in the face of the procedures that are performed to restore normal disc-condyle relationships. It should be understood that successful surgical outcome of any temporomandibular joint procedure is going to be based on eliminating the etiological, contributing, and perpetuating factors that are responsible for the disease and localized dysfunction of the joint. Elimination of adverse loading to the joint and post-surgical range of motion exercises is of primary importance in the successful outcome of any surgical procedure of the temporomandibular joint.

References

1   Ohnishi M. Arthroscopy of the temporomandibular joint. J Jpn Stomatol Soc 1975; 42:207
2   Kino K. Morphological and structural observation of the synovial membranes and their folds relating to endoscopic findings in the upper cavity of the human temporomandibular joint. J Jpn Stomatol Soc 1980; 47:98
3   Murakami K, Ito K. Arthroscopy of the temporomandibular joint. In: Watanabe M (ed). Arthroscopy of small joints. Tokyo: Igaka, 1985; 128
4   Holmlund A, Hellsing G. Arthroscopy of the temporomandibular joint. An autopsy study. Int J Oral Maxillofac Surg 1985; 14:169
5   Moses J, Sartoris D, Glass G, et al. The effect of arthroscopic surgical lysis and lavage of the superior joint space of the TMJ on disc position and mobility. J Oral Maxillofac Surg 1989; 47:674
6   Gabler MJ, Greene CH, Palacios E, Perry HT. Effect of arthroscopic temporomandibular joint surgery on articular disc position. J Craniomandib Disord Facial Oral Pain 1989; 3:191
7   Montgomery MT, van Sickels J, Harms S, et al. Arthroscopic TMJ surgery: effects on signs, symptoms, and disc position. J Oral Maxillofac Surg 1989; 47:1263
8   Segami N, Murakami K, Iizuka T. Arthrographic evaluation of disc position following mandibular manipulation technique for internal derangement with closed lock of the temporomandibular joint. J Craniomandib Disord Facial Oral Pain 1990; 4:99
9   Sanders B. Arthroscopic surgery of the temporomandibular joint: treatment of internal derangement with persistent closed lock. Oral Surg Oral Med Oral Pathol 1986; 62:361
10 Ghadially FN, Roy S. Ultrastructure of synovial joints in health and disease. New York: Appleton Century, 1969
11 Swann DA, Radin EL, Nazmiec M, et al. Role of hyaluronic acid in joint lubrication. Ann Rheum Dis 1974; 33:318
12 Swann DA, Radin EL. The molecular basis of articular lubrication. I. Purification and properties of a lubricating fraction from bovine synovial fluid. J Biol Chem 1972; 274:8069
13 Jimenez SA. The connective tissue: structure, function, and metabolism. In: Schumacher HR (ed). Primer on the rheumatic diseases. 9th ed. Atlanta: Arthritis foundation, 1988; 6
14 Howell DS, Manicourt DH. Complex polysaccharides. In: Schumacher HR (ed). Primer on the rheumatic diseases. 9th ed. Atlanta: Arthritis foundation, 1988; 15
15 Dinarello CA. Interleukin-1 and the pathogenesis of the acute-phase response. N Engl J Med 1984; 311:1413

16 Gowen M, Wood DP, Ihrie EJ, et al. Stimulation by human interleukin-1 of cartilage breakdown and production of collagenase and proteoglycanase by human chondrocytes but not by human osteoblasts in vitro. Biochem Biophys Acta 1984; 797:186

17 Martel-Pelletier J, Pelletier JP, Malemud CJ. Activation of neutral metalloprotease in human osteoarthritic knee cartilage: evidence for degradation in the core protein of sulfated proteoglycan. Ann Rheum Dis 1988; 47:801

18 McCord JM. Oxygen-derived radicals: a link between reperfusion injury and inflammation. Ped Proc 1987; 46:2402

19 Merry P, Williams R, Cox N, et al. Comparative study of intra-articular pressure dynamics in joints with acute traumatic and chronic inflammatory effusions. Potential implications for hypoxic-reperfusion injury. Ann Rheum Dis 1991; 50:917

20 Nitzan DW. Intra-articular pressure in the functioning human temporomandibular joint and its alteration by uniform elevation of occlusal plane. J Oral Maxillofac Surg 1994; 52:671

21 Schwartz RD. Pathophysiology of temporomandibular disorders. In: Thomas M, Bronstein S (eds). Arthroscopy of the temporomandibular joint. Philadelphia: Saunders, 1991; 36

22 Radin EL, Paul IC, Rose M. Osteoarthritis as a final common pathway. In: Nuki G (ed). The etiopathogenesis of osteoarthritis. London: Pitman Medical, 1980; 84

23 de Bont LGM, Stegenga B, Boering G. Hard tissue pathology. Osteoarthrosis. In: Thomas M, Bronstein S (eds). Arthroscopy of the temporomandibular joint. Philadelphia: Saunders, 1991; 258

24 Radin EL. Biomechanical considerations. In: Moskowitz RW, Howell DS, Goldberg VM, et al. (eds). Osteoarthritis: diagnosis and management. Philadelphia: Saunders, 1984; 93

25 Barrett AJ, Saklatvala J. Proteinases in joint disease. In: Kelly WN, Harris ED jr, Ruddy S, Sledge CB (eds). Textbook of rheumatology. Philadelphia: Saunders, 1985

26 Hamerman D, Klagsbrun M. Osteoarthritis: emerging evidence for cell interactions in the breakdown and remodeling of cartilage. Am J Med 1985; 78:495

27 Hamerman D. The biology of osteoarthritis. N Engl J Med 1989; 320:1322

28 Stegenga B, de Bont LGM, Boering G. Osteoarthrosis as the cause of craniomandibular pain and dysfunction: a unifying concept. J Oral Maxillofac Surg 1989; 47:249

29 Israel HA, Saed-Nejad, Ratcliff A. Early diagnosis of osteoarthrosis of the temporomandibular joint: correlation between arthroscopic diagnosis and keratin sulfate levels in synovial fluid. J Oral Maxillofac Surg 1991; 49:708

30 Quinn J, Bazan N. Identification of prostaglandin E and leukotriene B in the synovial fluid of painful, dysfunctional temporomandibular joints. J Oral Maxillofac Surg 1990; 48:968

31 Shafer DM, Assael L, White LB, Rossomando EF. Tumor necrosis factor as a biochemical marker of pain and outcome in temporomandibular joints with internal derangements. J Oral Maxillofac Surg 1994; 52:786

32 Israel HA, Ellis P, Furgang D. Synovial fluid protein concentration in patients undergoing temporomandibular joint arthroscopy. J Dent Res 1990; 69:296

33 Nitzan DW, Dolwick MF. An alternative explanation for the genesis of closed-lock symptoms in the internal derangement process. J Oral Maxillofac Surg 1991; 49:810

34 Nitzan DW, Dolwick MF, Martinez GA. Temporomandibular joint arthrocentesis: a simplified treatment for severe limited mouth opening. J Oral Maxillofac Surg 1991; 48:1163

35 Scapino RP. Histopathology associated with malposition of human temporomandibular disc. Oral Surg Oral Med Oral Pathol 1983; 59:382

36 Bibb C, Pullinger A. The histologic basis and clinical implications for temporomandibular joint adaptation. In: Clark GT, Sanders B, Bertolami C (eds). Diagnostic and surgical arthroscopy of the temporomandibular joint. Philadelphia: Saunders, 1993; 117

37 Sanders B, Buoncristiani R. A 5 year experience with arthroscopic lysis and lavage for treatment of painful temporomandibular joint hypomobility. In: Clark GT, Sanders B, Bertolami CN (eds). Advances in diagnostic and surgical arthroscopy of the temporomandibular joint. Philadelphia: Saunders, 1993; 31

38 Moses JJ, Poker ID. Temporomandibular joint arthroscopy: the endaural approach. Int J Oral Surg 1989; 18:347

39 White R. Retrospective analysis of 100 consecutive surgical arthroscopies of the temporomandibular joint. J Oral Maxillofac Surg 1989; 47:1014

40 Indresano TA. Arthroscopic surgery of the temporomandibular joint: report of 64 patients with long term follow-up. J Oral Maxillofac Surg 1989; 47:439

41 Israel HA, Roser S. Patient response to temporomandibular arthroscopy: preliminary findings in 24 patients. J Oral Maxillofac Surg 1989; 47:570

42 Nitzan DW, Dolwick MF, Heft MW. Arthroscopic lavage and lysis of the temporomandibular joint: a change in perspective. J Oral Maxillofac Surg 1990; 48:798

43 Perrott DH, Alborz A, Kaban LB, Helms CA. A prospective evaluation of the effectiveness of temporomandibular joint arthroscopy. J Oral Maxillofac Surg 1990; 48:1029

44 Clark GT, Liu C. Arthroscopic treatment of the human temporomandibular joint. In: Clark GT, Sanders B, Bertolami CN (eds). Advances in diagnostic and surgical arthroscopy of the temporomandibular joint. Philadelphia: Saunders, 1993; 85

45 Davis CL, Kaminishi RM, Marshall MW. Arthroscopic surgery for treatment of closed-lock. J Oral Maxillofac Surg 1991; 49:704

46 Moore LJ. Arthroscopic surgery for the treatment of restrictive temporomandibular joint disease. A prospective longitudinal study. In: Clark GT, Sanders B, Bertolami CN (eds). Advances in diagnostic and surgical arthroscopy of the temporomandibular joint. Philadelphia: Saunders, 1993; 35

47 Zeitler DL, Porter BT. A retrospective study comparing arthroscopic surgery with arthrotomy and disc repositioning. In: Clark GT, Sanders B, Bertolami CN (eds). Advances in diagnostic and surgical arthroscopy of the temporomandibular joint. Philadelphia: Saunders, 1993; 47

48 Stegenga B. Temporomandibular joint osteoarthrosis and internal derangement. Diagnostic and therapeutic outcome assessment. Thesis, University of Groningen, The Netherlands, 1991

Management of Temporomandibular
Joint Degenerative Diseases
ed. by B. Stegenga & L.G.M. de Bont
© 1996 Birkhäuser Verlag Basel/Switzerland

Biologic basis for modified condylotomy in the management of temporomandibular joint degenerative diseases

Samuel J. McKenna

Department of Oral and Maxillofacial Surgery, School of Medicine, Vanderbilt University, Nashville, Tennessee 37232, USA

Summary: The biologic basis for treating temporomandibular joint internal derangement with modified condylotomy rests in the ability of this procedure to improve or normalize disc position and favorably alter the course of osteoarthrosis and internal derangement. Data presented here favor modified condylotomy over other disc-preserving treatments for temporomandibular joint internal derangement.

Introduction

Condylotomy, though described over thirty years ago,[1,2] has gained little recognition for the treatment of temporomandibular joint disorders. Nickerson is credited with the introduction of a number of important technical modifications of the original closed condylotomy, and he renamed the changed operation the modified condylotomy.[3] In spite of several early reports describing successful management of temporomandibular joint internal derangement,[4-7] condylotomy has not gained popularity among American surgeons. The purpose of this chapter is to review current information regarding modified condylotomy, and to discuss the biologic basis and practical considerations regarding the use of this treatment in the management of temporomandibular joint internal derangements.

Biologic basis for modified condylotomy

The biologic basis for any treatment is founded on a scientifically rational explanation for the effect(s) of identifiable components of the treatment. Most treatments for symptomatic temporomandibular joint internal derangement have been directed toward relief of pain and mechanical symptoms. The observation that not all joints with internal derangement are painful,[8,9] and that some treatments for internal derangements seem to eliminate pain without improving disc position,[10-12] has brought into question the importance of disc position in the pathogenesis and treatment of temporomandibular joint pain. Though restoration of normal disc position may not always be required for pain relief, doing so may increase the likelihood of pain relief.[13-15] Further evidence suggests that in patients with a painful reducing disc displacement, symptoms can be controlled by normalization of the disc-condyle relationship and symptoms may recur with return to the displaced disc status.[16] Most treatments for internal derangement are composed of more than one potentially therapeutic component. Condylotomy, for example, may alter pain by increasing the joint space independent of any change in disc position. Only controlled studies will clarify the role of various treatments in the modulation of joint pain.

Any discussion regarding the biologic basis of a treatment must take into consideration the natural course of the disorder being treated. The progressive nature of internal derangement has been demonstrated.[8,17] Regressive remodeling of the condyle and fossa, when it occurs, is almost always associated with permanent disc displacement. A number of reports have established a relationship between disc displacement, osteoarthrosis, and skeletal jaw deformity.[8,17-21] Skeletal jaw deformity in the growing individual with an internal derangement may result from regressive condylar remodeling but also from deficient mandibular growth. Based on these observations, it would appear that disc position is important. Therefore, if disc position can be improved, the biologic basis of modified condylotomy is to alter favorably the course of temporomandibular joint internal derangement and osteoarthrosis, especially to reverse it.

Modified condylotomy is the only surgical procedure that has been demonstrated to frequently re-establish a normal disc-condyle relationship.[3,13,22] One of the early pioneers in the development of the closed condylotomy hypothesized that surgical forward positioning of the condyle, as in a displaced condylar fracture, would allow normalization of a deranged disc-condyle relationship.[5] He further noted that there was a positive correlation between the patient's report of improved symptoms and increased joint space on post-operative radiographs. Nickerson and Veaco, applying the modified condylotomy to joints with reducing disc displacement, were the first to image disc position after condylotomy.[3] At a mean of 66 months following surgery, arthrograms of ten joints revealed a normal disc-condyle relationship in four joints and improved disc position in three joints. Plain radiographs revealed no regressive remodeling. Subsequently, Nickerson reported normalization and improvement of disc position in 63% and 20%, respectively, in 64 joints with reducing disc displacement, an average of 2.6 years following modified condylotomy.[22] There was no osteoarthrotic deformation in any joint with normal disc position. Seven of 64 joints progressed to permanent disc displacement at some point after condylotomy but regressive remodeling occurred in only two of these joints. Importantly, 23% of the joints in this study had progressed to permanent disc displacement shortly before being unlocked at the time of condylotomy. The incidence of progression of reducing to permanent disc displacement and osteoarthrosis in this report is substantially less than what would be predicted based on our present knowledge of the natural history of internal derangement and osteoarthrosis.[8,17,23]

Hall et al. reported a normal disc-condyle relationship in 95% of 19 joints imaged with magnetic resonance imaging, an average of 26 months following modified condylotomy for reducing disc displacement.[24] More recently, Werther et al. have evaluated disc position by magnetic resonance imaging in 80 joints, one to fourteen days following modified condylotomy for painful reducing disc displacement.[25] Overall, disc position was normal in 78%, improved in 15% and unchanged in 7% of joints. When pre-operative disc displacement was classified according to five configurations, normalization of disc position was most common with medial (100%), anterior (82%) and medial-rotary (87%) displacements. Importantly, these three configurations accounted for 77% of the disc diagnosis. Anterior-lateral and anterior-medial displacements were normalized in 55% and 40% of joints, respectively. However, these two latter configurations accounted for only 17% of disc diagnoses prior to surgery. Recently, magnetic resonance images have been reviewed of 17 joints an average of 9.8 years following condylotomy for symptomatic reducing and permanent disc displacement that could be unlocked at the time of condylotomy. Disc position was determined to be normal, reducing and permanently displaced in 59%, 29% and 12% of joints, respectively. Follow-up plain radiographs were not obtained in this unpublished study, but with the exception of one joint with normal disc position and slight degenerative changes, there was no regressive remodeling by T1 and T2 weighted magnetic resonance images. These data on disc position compare favorably with Nickerson's earlier arthrographic data from the same population of patients approximately three years after modified condylotomy.[22] The incidence of progression of reducing to permanent disc displacement is substantially better than what would be predicted from recent data describing cessation of clicking after two to four years in 34% of joints with reducing discs that only received supportive treatments.[23] The apparent small decrease in joints with normal disc position nearly ten years following condylotomy suggests some tendency for recurrence of internal derangement. As the initiating events of internal derangement are largely unknown,[8,17] it is conceivable that, after nearly ten years of function, some treated joints with normal disc position may again be subject to the development of an internal derangement. The low incidence of radiographically visible osteoarthrosis ten years following condylotomy is consistent with reports that condylotomy may limit the progression of internal derangement and osteoarthrosis.[3,22,24]

Comparison of these data with disc imaging after arthroscopy[11,12,26] and arthrotomy[10,27,28] demonstrate a superior ability of modified condylotomy to normalize disc position. Published data on disc imaging before and after treatment of internal derangement with mandibular repositioning appliances are limited.[13,29,30] Although repositioning appliance therapy may normalize disc position,[13,30] the extent of dental treatments required to maintain the disc in a reduced position make this process less efficient than modified condylotomy.

The biologic basis of modified condylotomy is normalization or improvement of disc position that appears to alter favorably the natural course of internal derangement and osteoarthrosis. Although unstudied, the theoretical benefit of modified condylotomy in the growing individual with temporomandibular joint internal derangement is obvious. Another basis for modified condylotomy may be improvement in pain and other symptoms from increased joint space created by this operation.

Objectives of modified condylotomy

As with other treatments for internal derangement, the primary objectives of modified condylotomy are relief of pain and mechanical symptoms, and resumption of more normal jaw activity. The mechanical symptoms associated with recurrent mandibular luxation have also been successfully addressed with modified condylotomy.[4,31]

Limitations of modified condylotomy

Modified condylotomy has been used to treat joints with reducing disc displacement, and joints that have recently progressed to permanent disc displacement that can be unlocked at the time of condylotomy.[5,22,24] There are no reports to support the use of modified condylotomy for joints with a chronic permanent disc displacement without active osteoarthritis. However, in an unpublished study by Hall and Navarro, equivalent pain reduction has been demonstrated two, four and twelve months following modified condylotomy for reducing disc displacement (40 joints) and chronic permanent disc displacement (19 joints). Any benefit derived from modified condylotomy in this situation is not from improvement in disc position but from some other factor associated with the procedure (i.e., increased joint space).

With advancements in magnetic resonance technology, several variations of reducing disc displacements have been recognized. After a systematic review of magnetic resonance images before and one to fourteen days after modified condylotomy it has been noted that fewer reducing disc displacements had been corrected to normal disc position when the disc was displaced anteromedially or anterolaterally. In contrast, medial, anterior and medial-rotary type disc displacements frequently returned to normal position after modified condylotomy.[25] A biomechanical explanation for the different variations of reducing disc displacements is not known, but observed differences in disc reduction following modified condylotomy may have important clinical implications.

Closed condylotomy has been advocated for the treatment of active temporomandibular joint osteoarthrosis.[32,33] Although improvement in pain has been reported immediately after condylotomy, long-term resolution of symptoms as well as evidence of radiographic healing may relate more to the natural course of osteoarthrosis than to the treatment. Reports of modified condylotomy for the treatment of active osteoarthritis are limited.[34]

Occlusal change following modified condylotomy, although rare, is more likely to occur in the patient without good intercuspation of teeth before operation. Specifically, patients with cross bites and deficient centric occlusal contacts, especially on the side opposite the operation, in the case of a unilateral condylotomy, are at greater risk of experiencing some bite ambiguity after release of maxillo-mandibular fixation. Similarly, in patients with dentures, the occlusion may be difficult to control after modified condylotomy. These concerns for bite change may be more important with bilateral condylotomy.

Surgical technique

As originally described, condylotomy was a closed oblique subcondylar osteo- tomy.[4] Later, Nickerson performed the procedure transorally as a modification of the intraoral vertical ramus osteotomy.[3] The principal difference between modified condylotomy and intraoral vertical ramus osteotomy is the deliberate stripping of a portion of the medial pterygoid muscle from the distal aspect of the proximal segment to promote condylar sag (figure 1). Initially, the proximal segment was trimmed to allow for a small amount of overlap of the segments or for the creation of a butt joint (figures 2 and 3). The rationale for trimming the proximal segments was to allow for a slight amount of forward displacement of the condylar segment, presumably to a more normal position beneath the displaced disc. Subsequently, magnetic resonance imaging demonstrated that, under the influence of modified condylotomy, the disc will migrate posteriorly and assume a more normal relationship with the glenoid fossa and condyle.[24] Although most reports of modified condylotomy have described proximal segment trimming, it is possible that disc position can be normalized without

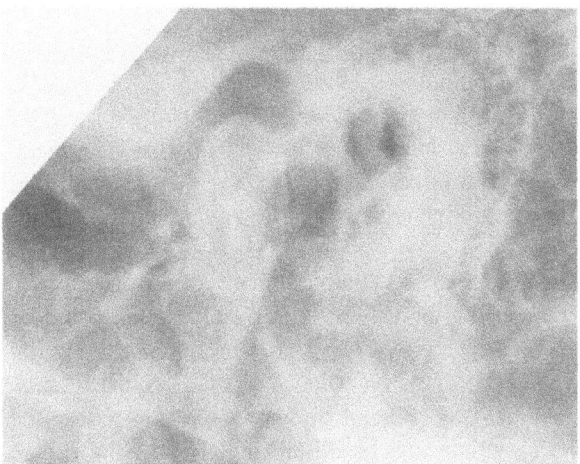

Figure 1.
Transcranial radiograph 24 hours after modified condy- lotomy, moderate condylar sag.

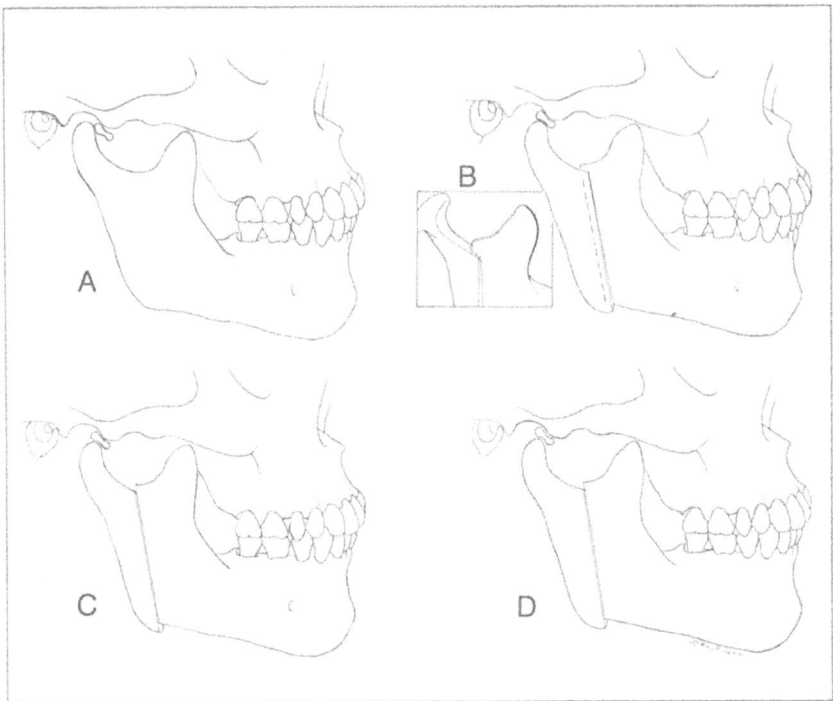

Figure 2.
Illustration of disc and condylar position after modified condylotomy.
A. Reducing disc displacement before operation.
B. Medial edge of proximal segment trimmed to allow lateral overlap. Downward and forward
   movement of condyle, backward movement of disc to superior position.
C. Same as B but entire leading edge of proximal segment trimmed, butt joint.
D. Proximal segment not trimmed, downward and minimal forward movement of condyle, butt joint.
   Backward movement of disc to superior position.

trimming. Rarely, the proximal segment will displace medially with a possible associated neurapraxia of the mandibular nerve. This problem can be largely prevented by judicious trimming of the proximal segment allowing for a slight amount of lateral overlap of the distal segment by the proximal segment. Through attempts to strip less (approximately 5.0 mm) medial pterygoid muscle, it appears that minimal condylar sag is required to affect disc repositioning.

As originally described,[3] the modified condylotomy was performed with the mouth propped open beyond the point where an opening click could be detected. The rationale for this manoeuvre was that, presumably, the entire procedure was performed with the disc in a reduced position. Subsequently, this step has been eliminated and no deliberate attempt is made to reduce the displaced disc. Data on disc position after modified condylotomy performed with the mouth open compare favorably with disc imaging data where the

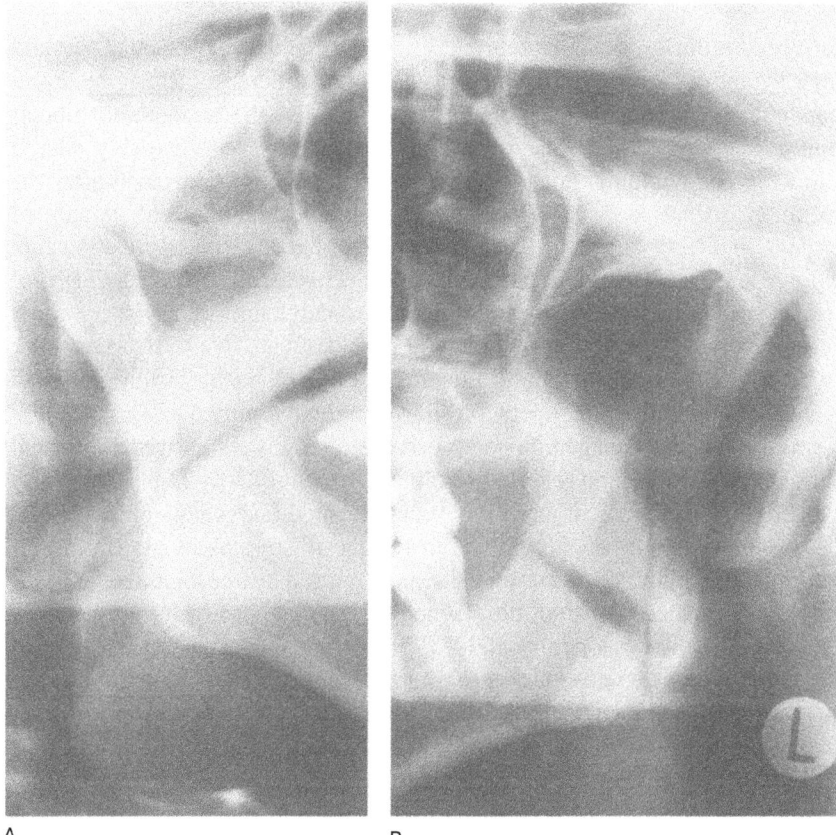

A   B

Figure 3.
Panoramic radiograph after modified condylotomy.
A. Medial edge of proximal segment trimmed, lateral overlap.
B. Proximal segment not trimmed, butt joint.

mouth has not been deliberately opened.[3,24] There does not appear to be any benefit to performing this surgery in the open mouth position.

A variable period of maxillo-mandibular fixation is employed with modified condylotomy, ranging from five weeks to as short as one week.[3,35] Current techniques utilize 2-3 weeks of maxillo-mandibular fixation followed by 3-4 weeks of continuous training elastic use. Active range of motion exercises are initiated following the release of maxillo-mandibular fixation to overcome the variable tendency for trismus after a mandibular osteotomy. Generally, arch bars are removed six to eight weeks following the operation. Bilateral surgery may require slightly longer periods of training elastic use for establishment of a stable occlusion. Modified condylotomy is generally performed on an outpatient basis without the necessity for overnight hospitalization.

Treatment outcome

Early reports of closed condylotomy describe successful management of pain and other symptoms associated with suspected internal derangement,[5-7] recurrent mandibular luxation,[4,31] and active osteoarthritis of the temporomandibular joint.[32,33] It was generally believed that disc position was favorably altered following condylotomy, however, disc imaging was not performed after the operation. Increased joint space seemed to be an important determinant of success,[5] indirectly suggesting some alteration of the disc-condyle relationship. More recent reports have described improvement in pain from reducing disc displacement at least 85% of the time after open condylotomy.[35-38] Nickerson and Veaco reported improved symptoms in 93% of patients five to six years after modified condylotomy for painful reducing disc displacement.[3] Arthrography an average of 66 months after operation showed normal or improved disc position in seven of ten joints imaged. No joints demonstrated any regressive remodeling. Subsequently, Nickerson reported resolution of pain in 80% of 64 joints with reducing disc displacement nearly four years after modified condylotomy. In 83%, disc position was normal or improved an average of 2.6 years after operation. Of the 12 painful joints, ten had normal disc position and in nine joints the pain was felt to be associated with night-time clenching. Although in nearly one quarter of the joints the disc was permanently displaced but unlockable at the time of operation, only seven of 64 joints became chronically displaced with two showing regressive remodeling. Others have reported frequent normalization or improvement in disc position following modified condylotomy (figure 4).[24]

Except possibly for discectomy, there are scant long-term data on any treatment for temporomandibular joint internal derangement. Recently, questionnaires were mailed to 39 patients an average of 9.8 years after modified condylotomy for symptomatic reducing disc displacement. Seventeen patients (27 joints) responded to this questionnaire and 12 patients (20 joints) agreed to return for clinical and magnetic resonance examination. Two patients (three joints) were not imaged because they underwent sagittal split osteotomy (one joint) or arthroscopy (two joints) prior to the follow-up visit. Only eleven joints (41%) were pain-free but in the remainder, pain was rated four or less on a scale of ten except in three joints. All but one of these patients described daytime and/or nighttime parafunctional jaw activity. Sixty-nine percent of the patients had an unrestricted diet and no patient was limited to soft or liquid foods. Sixty-five percent of the joints examined were non-tender. The mean interincisal opening was 44.8 mm, a 2.1 mm decrease from before condylotomy. Importantly, the maximum interincisal opening measured before condylotomy was under general anesthesia. Magnetic resonance imaging revealed normal disc position in 59%, reducing discs in 29%, and permanently displaced discs in 12% of joints (figure 5). Modified condylotomy was described as tremendously helpful in 75%, somewhat helpful in 17%, and without effect in 8% of joints. Eighty-seven percent of patients affirmed that they would willingly undergo modified condylotomy again, if necessary.

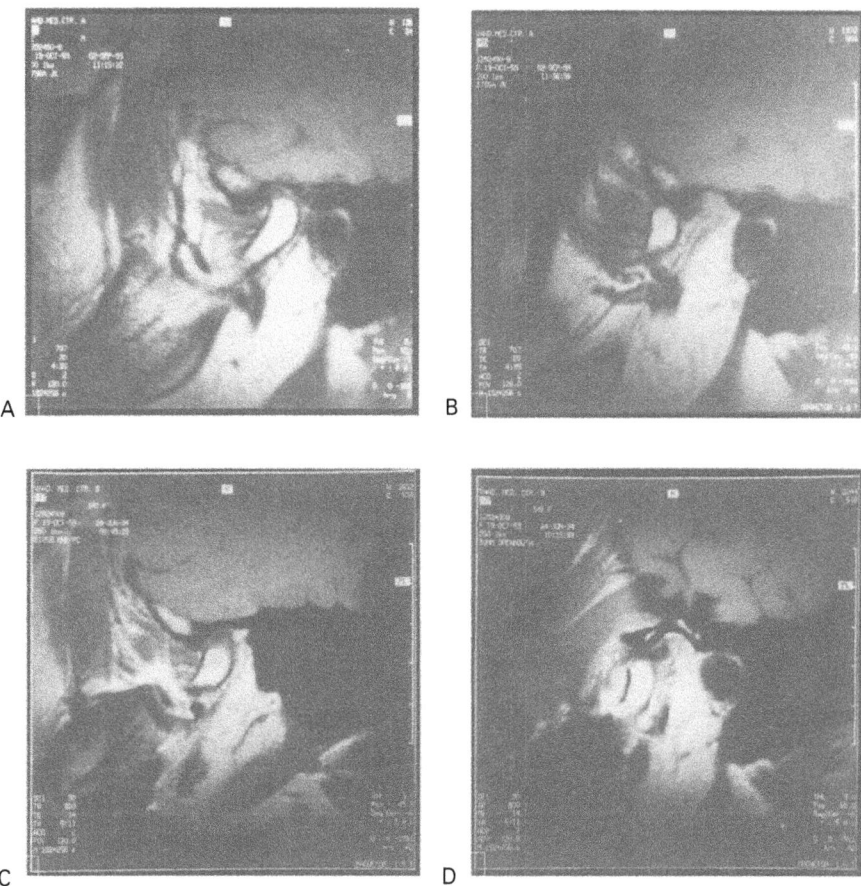

Figure 4.
T1 weighted magnetic resonance image before and after condylotomy for reducing disc displacement.
A. Closed mouth image depicting anterior displacement before condylotomy.
B. Open mouth image before operation showing disc reduction.
C. Closed mouth view 9 months after modified condylotomy, normal disc position.
D. Open mouth view 9 months after modified condylotomy, satisfactory condylar and disc mobility.

Current role for modified condylotomy

The current role for modified condylotomy is the management of pain, mechanical symptoms, or both caused by temporomandibular joint internal derangement. The ability of modified condylotomy to reverse reducing disc
displacement and its associated symptoms has been well demonstrated.[3,22,24]
Other reports suggest a role for modified condylotomy in the management of
pain with an active osteoarthritis.[32,33] Unpublished data to support the use of
modified condylotomy in joints with chronic permanent disc displacement
without active osteoarthritis suggest a possible new application of this proce-

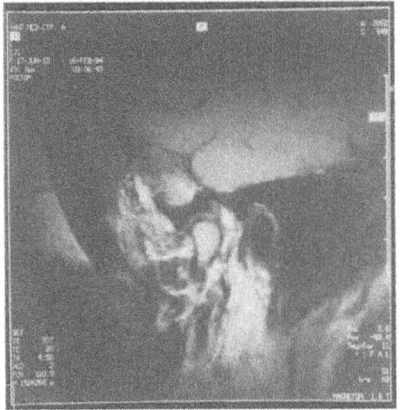 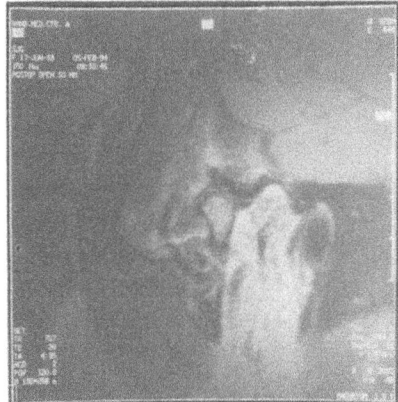

A   B

Figure 5.
T1 weighted magnetic resonance image nearly
10 years after modified condylotomy for reduc-
ing disc displacement.
A. Closed mouth image, normal disc position.
B. Open mouth image, satisfactory disc mobility.
C. Closed mouth coronal image, normal disc
   position.

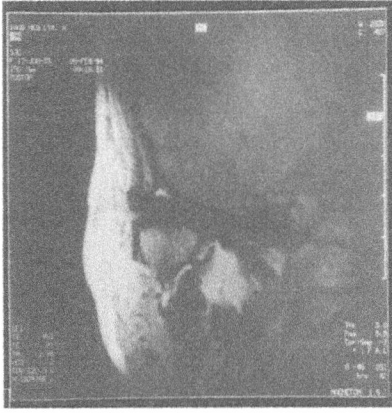

C

dure. Finally, earlier favorable results following treatment of recurrent luxation
with closed condylotomy support a role for modified condylotomy in the
management of this problem.[31]

Future perspectives

Support for any treatment for internal derangement of the temporomandibular
joint should be based on controlled studies demonstrating a treatment effect.
Through as yet incompletely understood adaptive mechanisms, symptoms of
internal derangement and/or osteoarthrosis tend to improve over a period of
two to four years without any treatment.[23] Any claim to long-term treatment
success may in part be accounted for by the natural tendency for spontaneous
improvement or resolution of symptoms associated with osteoarthrosis and
internal derangement. Controlled studies are needed to clarify the therapeutic
component(s) of various treatments employed today. Further, the merits of a

particular treatment should be evaluated by the ability of the treatment to favorably alter the course of the disorder. Since not all configurations of reducing disc displacement seem to be normalized or improved to the same degree following modified condylotomy, studies of patient response as a function of the type of disc displacement are needed.

Not all temporomandibular joint internal derangements are painful.[8,9] Furthermore, relief of pain can occur with treatments that do not alter disc position,[10-12] suggesting that factors other than disc position may be important. This apparent paradox may be explained by adjustments in jaw function and loading imposed by many surgical and non-surgical treatments. Similarly, long-term improvement in symptoms may result from a patient's effort to moderate joint loading and from the potential for the mandibular locomotor apparatus to adapt. Disc displacement, however, seems to be important in the development of skeletal jaw deformity from osteoarthrosis and/or from defective mandibular growth. Modified condylotomy appears to have the ability to restage early internal derangement and decrease the frequency of progressive osteoarthrosis below that which would be expected with only supportive treatment.[3,22,24] Studies to clarify a possible role for modified condylotomy in the prevention of skeletal jaw deformity are needed.

Treatment of chronic permanent disc displacement with modified condylotomy is directed towards relief of pain and not towards normalization of disc position. The basis for any early resolution of symptoms in this situation is likely secondary to increased joint space. It is not known whether this application of modified condylotomy will delay or prevent progression of osteoarthrosis as has been observed when a reducing disc displacement is managed with modified condylotomy. It is possible that modified condylotomy may enhance the adaptive capacity of the chronically deranged joint, leading to early resolution or improvement of symptoms. Condylotomy may, as suggested by Nickerson,[39] favorably influence the course of osteoarthrosis by the well recognized though inconsistent process of progressive remodeling. Further studies to define the role of modified condylotomy in the management of the chronically displaced disc are needed.

Summary and conclusions

Condylotomy is the only surgical treatment for temporomandibular joint internal derangement that frequently normalizes disc position. Immediate and long-term improvement in pain and mechanical symptoms associated with internal derangement occurs in a high percentage of patients. The biologic basis for modified condylotomy rests in the ability of this procedure to favorably alter the natural course of osteoarthrosis and internal derangement. With the possible exception of discectomy,[40] no other treatment for internal derangement has been demonstrated to affect the course of osteoarthrosis. This has interesting implications for the prevention of skeletal deformity both from regressive remodeling and, in the growing individual, from deficient mandibular growth. Preliminary long-term data on modified condylotomy show that protection from progression of osteoarthrosis, though not perfect, seems to be a lasting benefit from this treatment. That some joints, presumably with normal disc position immediately following modified condylotomy, show a reducing disc ten years after the operation does not detract from the value of this procedure. Such cases represent "new" internal derangements caused by certain yet unknown initiating events. Although many questions remain to be answered by future studies, there is a sound basis evolved to support the use of modified condylotomy in the management of symptomatic internal derangement of the temporomandibular joint.

Acknowledgements

I wish to thank James W. Nickerson, Jr., DMD, and H. David Hall, DMD, MD, for their constructive criticism of this manuscript.

References

1 Staz J. The treatment of disturbance of the temporomandibular articulation. J Dent Assoc of South Africa 1952; 6:324

2 Ward TG, Smith DG, Sommar M. Condylotomy for mandibular joints. Br Dent J 1957; 103:147

3 Nickerson JW Jr, Veaco WS. Condylotomy in surgery of the temporomandibular joint. Oral Maxillofac Surg Clin of North Am 1989; 1:303

4 Ward TG. Surgery of the mandibular joint. Ann R Coll Surg Engl 1961; 28:139

5 Campbell W. Clinical radiological investigations of the mandibular joints. Br J Radiol 1965; 38:401

6 Banks P, Mackenzie I. Condylotomy, a clinical and experimental appraisal of a surgical technique. J Maxillofac Surg 1975; 3:170

7 Tasanen A, von Konow L. Closed condylotomy in the treatment of idiopathic and traumatic pain-dysfunction syndrome of the temporomandibular joint. Int J Oral Surg 1973; 2:102

8 Nickerson JW Jr, Boering G. Natural course of osteoarthrosis as it relates to internal derangement of the temporomandibular joint. Oral Maxillofac Surg Clin North Am 1989; 1:27

9 Westesson PL, Ericksson L. Reliability of a negative clinical temporomandibular joint examination: prevalence of disc displacement in asymptomatic temporomandibular joints. Oral Surg Oral Med Oral Pathol 1989; 68:551

10 Montgomery MT, Gordon SM, VanSickels JE, et al. Changes in signs and symptoms following temporomandibular joint disc repositioning surgery. J Oral Maxillofac Surg 1992; 50:320

11 Montgomery MT, VanSickels JE, Harms SE, et al. Arthroscopic TMJ surgery: effects on signs, symptoms and disc position. J Oral Maxillofac Surg 1989; 47:1263

12 Montgomery MT, VanSickels JE, Harms SE. Success of temporomandibular joint arthroscopy in disc displacement with and without reduction. Oral Surg Oral Med Oral Pathol 1991; 71:651

13 Westesson PL, Lundh H. Temporomandibular joint disc displacement: arthrographic and to-mographic follow-up after 6 months treatment with disc repositioning onlays. Oral Surg Oral Med Oral Pathol 1988; 66:271

14 Anderson GC, Schulte JK, Goodkind RJ. Comparative study of two treatment methods for internal derangement of the TMJ. J Prosthet Dent 1985; 53:393

15 Conway WF, Hayes CW, Campbell RL, et al. Temporomandibular joint after meniscoplasty – appearance at MR imaging. Radiol 1991; 180:749

16 Lundh H, Westesson PL, Jisander S, et al. Disc repositioning overlays in the treatment of

temporomandibular joint disc displacement: comparison with a flat occlusal splint and with no treatment. Oral Surg Oral Med Oral Pathol 1988; 66: 155

17 Boering G. Arthrosis deformans van het kaakgewricht. Thesis, University of Groningen, The Netherlands, 1966

18 Rickets RM. Clinical implications of the temporomandibular joint. Am J Orthod 1966; 52:416

19 Nickerson JW Jr, Moystad A. Observations of individuals with radiographic bilateral condylar remodeling. J Craniomandibular Pract 1982; 1:21

20 Link JJ, Nickerson JW. Temporomandibular joint internal derangement in an orthognathic population. Int J Adult Orthod Orthognath Surg 1992; 7:161

21 Schellhas KP, Keck RJ. Disorder of skeletal occlusion and temporomandibular joint disease. Northwest Dent 1989; 68:35

22 Nickerson JW Jr. The role of condylotomy in the mangement of temporomandibular joint disorders. In: Controversies in Oral and Maxillofacial Surgery, 4th ed. Worthington P, Evan J (eds). Philadelphia: Saunders, 1994; 339

23 de Leeuw R, Boering G, Stegenga B, et al. Clinical signs of TMJ osteoarthrosis and internal derangement 30 years after nonsurgical treatment. J Orofacial Pain 1994; 8:18

24 Hall HD, Nickerson JW Jr, McKenna SJ. Modified condylotomy for treatment of the painful temporomandibular joint with a reducing disc. J Oral Maxillofac Surg 1993; 51:133

25 Werther JR, Hall HD, Gibbs SJ. Disc position before and after modified condylotomy in 80 symptomatic temporomandibular joints. Oral Surg Oral Med Oral Pathol 1995; 79:668

26 Gabler MJ, Greene CS, Palacios E, et al. Effect of arthroscopic temporomandibular joint surgery on articular disc position. J Craniomandib Disord Facial Oral Pain 1989; 3:191

27 Westesson PL, Cohen JM, Tallents RH. Magnetic resonance imaging of temporomandibular joint after surgical treatment of internal derangement. Oral Surg Oral Med Oral Pathol 1991; 71:651

28 Conway WF, Hayes CW, Campbell RL, et al. Temporomandibular joint after meniscoplasty: appearance at MR imaging. Radiology 1991; 180:749

29 Kirk WS. Magnetic resonance imaging and tomographic evaluation of occlusal appliance treatment for advanced internal derangement of the temporomandibular joint. J Oral Maxillofac Surg 1991; 49:9

30 Lundh H, Westesson PL. Long-term follow-up occlusal treatment to correct abnormal temporomandibular joint disc position. Oral Surg Oral Med Oral Pathol 1989; 67:2

31 Tasanen A, Lamberg MA. Closed condylotomy in the treatment of recurrent dislocation of the mandibular condyle. Int J Oral Surg 1978; 7:1

32 Tasanen A, Lamberg MA. Closed condylotomy in the treatment of osteoarthrosis of the temporomandibular joint. Int J Oral Surg 1974; 3:102

33 Tasanen A, Jokinen J. Closed condylotomy in the treatment of osteoarthritis of the temporomandibular joint: clinical and radiographic study. Int J Oral Surg 1981; 10:239

34 Albury CA Jr. Progressive remodeling of an osteoarthritic condyle postoperative coronocondylotomy: a case report. J Craniomandibular Pract 1989; 7:245

35 Bell WH, Yamaguchi Y, Poor MR. Treatment of temporomandibular joint dysfunction by intraoral vertical ramus osteotomy. J Adult Orthodon Orthognath Surg 1990; 5:9

36 Upton LG, Sullivan SM. Modified condylotomies for management of mandibular prognathism and TMJ internal derangement. J Clin Orthod 1990; 24:697

37 Upton LG, Sullivan SM. The treatment of temporomandibular joint internal derangements using a modified open condylotomy: a preliminary report. J Oral Maxillofac Surg 1991; 49:578

38 Shevel E. Intra-oral condylotomy for the treatment of temporomandibular joint derangement. Int J Oral Maxillofac Surg 1991; 20:360

39 Nickerson JW Jr. The role of condylotomy for treating internal derangement of the temporomandibular joint. Oral Maxillofac Clin North Am 1994; 6:277

40 Wilkes CH. Surgical treatment of internal derangements of the temporomandibular joint: A long-term study. Arch Otolaryngol Head Neck Surg 1991; 117:64

Management of Temporomandibular
Joint Degenerative Diseases
ed. by B. Stegenga & L.G.M. de Bont
© 1996 Birkhäuser Verlag Basel/Switzerland

Temporomandibular joint disc surgery: biologic basis and treatment outcome

Doran E. Ryan

Department of Oral and Maxillofacial Surgery, Medical College of Wisconsin, Milwaukee, Wisconsin 53226, USA

Summary: Disc repair appears to have a biologic basis in Wilkes' stage II internal joint derangements. With proper patient selection and good surgical technique to stabilize the disc back to a normal relationship to the condyle, the long-term success is around 90%. Magnetic resonance imaging is the technique of choice for follow-up evaluation. Well-controlled studies are still needed to verify results.

Introduction

Disc repositioning is the oldest temporomandibular joint surgical procedure according to the world's English literature. The first known disc repair was by Annadale in 1887.[1] Behan described the second disc plication to correct a loose cartilage in the temporomandibular joint with locking.[2] He described this as a "posterior displacement of the meniscus and an inability of the patient to close her mouth all the way". No further literature described disc repair until the 1970s. Between the early 1900s and the 1970s, discectomy or high condylectomy was the surgical temporomandibular joint treatment of choice. In the 1950s and 1960s, because of failures and complications following surgical management in treating temporomandibular arthropathies, non-surgical therapy became the standard of care in many parts of the world.

A major event, which would in time renew interest in disc repair, was the description of the use of arthrography of the temporomandibular joint.[3] Wilkes re-emphasized the significance of arthrography as an effective means to visualize the integrity and position of the disc, thereby defining the pathophysiology of internal derangements.[4] McCarty and Farrar clearly described a disc repair procedure which would become a standard.[5] McCarty's initial surgical procedure included removal of a portion of the posterior attachment, repositioning the disc in a more posterior anatomical position, and reattaching the disc to the retrodiscal tissue. Arthroplasty of the posterior aspect of the condyle allowed correction of internal derangements without modifying the occlusion.

Biologic basis for disc surgery

Six topics need to be addressed, based on the available literature, to provide a basis for a possible biologic basis for disc repair surgery or for the need for further research efforts, i.e.,

- the function of the disc
- the objectives of disc surgery
- the normal anatomy of the temporomandibular joint soft tissues
- changes in the soft tissues with disc displacements
- progressiveness of changes
- the best time to accomplish corrective surgery for these displacements.

Function of the disc

Little scientific evidence is available to prove the true function of the disc, but based on the anatomical structures of the soft tissues of the temporomandibular joints, several theories have been presented.[6,7] A disc which is made up of fibrous tissue and positioned between two bony structures may serve as a shock absorber system during function. Since both the condyle and the articular eminence are convex surfaces, the general shape of the disc improves the fit between these bony surfaces and allows for smoother function. This would also help distribute the forces within the joint over a broader base. Synovial fluid appears to be essential for smooth function and nutrition of the joint surfaces. The movement of the disc between the bony surfaces appears to help spread the synovial fluid to all areas of the joint and across the articulating surfaces. The disc separates the joint into two joint spaces which allows for greater range of motion with rotation taking place in the inferior space and translation taking place in the superior joint space.

Objectives of disc repair surgery

If the articular disc of the temporomandibular joint has the functions previously described and has become displaced in an anterior or anterior-medial direction, the functions of the disc have been altered. The ultimate objective of this surgery would be to reposition the disc back to its normal relationship to the condyle and articular eminence, in this way restoring the normal anatomy and function of the joint. If pain and breakdown of the joint tissues is secondary to displacement and dysfunction of the disc along with pressure on innervated tissues and increased wear of articulating surfaces, then restoration of the normal anatomy should improve function, reduce pain, and prevent further damage to the soft and hard tissues of the joint.

Normal anatomy of the temporomandibular joint soft tissues

Articular disc

Macroscopically, the disc is made up of dense fibrous tissue that is concave on its inferior surface and saddle shaped on its superior surface with three distinct bands or zones.[8] The normal position of the disc with the mouth closed finds the posterior band of the disc over the superior aspect of the condyle, the intermediate band anterior-superior to the condyle and posterior-inferior to the eminence, and the anterior band just anterior to the condyle.

The microscopic anatomy of the disc has been well described.[9] The disc is composed of fibrous tissue which is avascular and non-innervated. It is able to flex which helps accommodate to the various shapes of the articulating surfaces of both the eminence and condyle. The general orientation of the fibers of the disc are in an anterior-posterior direction from its anterior attachment back to the posterior attachment. The intermediate zone has fiber orientation only in an anterior-posterior direction while the anterior and posterior bands also have intermingled transverse fibers.

Retrodiscal tissue

The retrodiscal tissue has been well described by several authors.[8-12] The retrodiscal tissue is divided into a superior lamina and an inferior lamina with a neurovascular zone in between. The superior lamina attaches posteriorly to the posterior wall of the glenoid fossa, i.e., the posterior glenoid process. The inferior lamina attaches to the posterior aspect of the condyle below the fibrocartilaginous covering. The superior lamina is made up of loose fibrous and fibro-elastic tissue, whereas the inferior lamina is composed of compact inelastic sheets of collagen fibers. Between the two layers is found the neurovascular zone containing numerous vascular channels and nerve fibers mainly from the auriculotemporal nerve and also small amounts of fat. The fibers of both the superior and inferior lamina splay out to become interlaced with the transverse fibers of the posterior band and also with the anterior-posterior fibers from the intermediate zone. The retrodiscal tissue is lined by synovial membrane.

Capsule

The joint capsule, as described by Boering,[13] consists of two main layers. The outer layer is fibrous tissue which posteriorly blends with the retrodiscal tissue and anteriorly with the anterior attachments of the disc and the superior belly of the lateral pterygoid muscle. The medial fibers are very loose and weak in nature, whereas the lateral capsule is strengthened by the temporomandibular ligament and is very inelastic. The inner layer of the capsule consists of loosely folded synovial membrane which lines all surfaces of the joint except the articulating surfaces. The capsule is highly innervated in all areas with free nerve endings derived from the auriculotemporal nerve in the posterior two-thirds of the capsule and the posterior deep temporal and masseteric nerves in the anterior one-third of the capsule.

Changes in soft tissues with disc displacement

Articular disc

Macroscopically the disc is described as being displaced in an anterior or anterior-medial direction. The posterior band of the disc would be located anterior to the condyle when the mouth is closed with the intermediate band at the inferior aspect of the articular eminence or even further forward. Kurita et al. and Scapino describe the thickening of the posterior band of the disc with disc displacement.[9,14] They also note a loss in anterior-posterior length of the disc which tends to become worse with more severe displacements. Heffez et al. describe changes in the normal morphology of the disc including changes in the lateral-medial dimension which they felt was secondary to squeezing the disc into a smaller joint space area medially and anteriorly to the condyle.[15] Westesson et al. and Luder agree with loss of the normal morphology with disc displacements and describe the loss of concavity on the inferior surface and the loss of the saddle shape on its superior surface.[16,17] Westesson et al. also describe the shortening of the disc especially in the anterior band of the disc.[16] Scapino describes flexure of the disc with displacement with either an upward or downward bend at the intermediate zone.[9] There is not a predominance of flexure in either direction.

Microscopic description of the disc when displaced shows loss of fiber orientation with transverse fibers found in the intermediate band causing disruption of the normal compact anterior-posterior fiber orientation. At the flexure of the disc as previously described, the fibers become oriented perpendicular to the surface.[9,17,18] Kurita et al., and Chase and McCoy describe cartilaginous and osseous metaplasia of the disc along with interstitial hyalinization. Other findings include proliferation of vessels into the non-vascular disc which are usually found anterior of the posterior band and on the inferior surface of the disc.[14,19] Degeneration of the disc, including basophilic and myxomatous degeneration along with loss of mean density of fibroblasts in the center of the disc have also been described.[14,17,18] Isacsson et al. note proliferation of connective tissue on the inferior-anterior part of the thickened posterior band.[18]

Retrodiscal tissue

The macroscopic changes of the retrodiscal tissue are well described by Scapino and Isacsson et al.[9,18] The retrodiscal tissue is divided into an anterior and posterior part once the disc has been displaced. The posterior part tends to migrate its posterior attachments both superiorly and anteriorly with the superior lamina migrating as far forward as the posterior slope of the articular eminence. The inferior lamina tends to migrate superiorly along the posterior aspect to the condyle. Significant changes are noted in the anterior part of the retrodiscal tissue which has now become the articulating surface between the condyle and the articular eminence. This portion becomes fibrotic, thin, and has demonstrated perforations at the junction between the retrodiscal tissue and the posterior band of the disc. Microscopically, the posterior part of the retrodiscal tissue shows increased vascularization, perivascular hyalinization, and vasodilatation with very little inflammation. The anterior part shows conversion to fibrocartilage, especially in younger individuals, loss of elastin, dysplastic cartilage especially in long-standing displacement, and surface fibrin the function of which is unknown. Essentially the anterior part of the retrodiscal tissue undergoes metaplasia toward the anatomical structure of the articulating disc, but over time the metaplasia can continue to cartilage or tissue can show degeneration and possible perforation.[9,14,17,19,20]

Capsule
The pathological changes noted in the capsule with displacement of the disc include hyperplasia of the synovial tissues along with edema, atrophy, and fibroid necrosis.[19] Chronic inflammatory cells are noted throughout the capsule and soft tissues of the joint but not in great numbers. The lateral recess of the capsule is displaced along with the disc and the capsule appears to adhere to the intermediate zone of the disc in many cases. The literature is very clear in demonstrating that permanent changes do take place in the soft tissues of the joint with displacement of the disc.

Disc displacement as a progressive disease

A reducing disc displacement appears to be progressive in many individuals but overall its course is unpredictable. Westesson and Lundh found that 20% of the individuals they studied went from an anterior displacement with reduction to a locked disc within a six month period.[21] Chase and McCoy demonstrated progressive metaplasia with age and with degree of disc displacement.[19] The findings were based on histologic evaluation of surgical specimens. Hall et al. found loss of elastin in the retrodiscal tissue with increasing age.[20] This change in elastin content was also found as the degree of displacement increased. Wilkes followed a group of non-surgically treated dislocated disc patients over 8.1 years and found a progressive change in their staging of disc displacements in 73.5%.[22] In an evaluation of autopsy specimens of younger and older individuals, Luder described a progressive remodeling in individuals under 20 and a regressive remodeling in individuals over 20.[17] He found that the displacements of the disc became more severe with age.

The inability to create an animal model with an anterior displaced disc has diminished the knowledge ascertained from animal studies. Most of the animal studies use normal disc positions as the baseline and then surgical procedures accomplished with follow-up evaluation of the results. Hall et al. did several procedures on monkeys, including disc repairs alone and disc repairs with bone surgery combined, and found that adhesions are a risk in these procedures especially when bone surgery is included.[23] The area of disc repair in the retrodiscal tissue tended to adhere to either the area of condyloplasty or eminoplasty. Eppley et al. used a rabbit model to investigate where the incision should be placed in the soft tissues of the disc or the retrodiscal tissue to effect the best healing.[24] They determined that the incision needed to be in vascularized tissue for the healing to take place. Disc tissue would not heal to disc tissue and the retrodiscal tissue would not heal back to avascular disc tissue. McDonald found that doing discectomies on rats would change the form of the condyle as they developed and concluded that the disc directs the form of the condyle.[25] If a perforation is made in the disc of a sheep, it will not repair itself.[26] Ali et al. created an internal joint derangement model in rabbits and then evaluated histological changes seen over time.[27] Fiber orientation of the disc and retrodiscal tissue would change over time with internal derangements. These findings certainly agree with the autopsy findings of other authors.

The best time to accomplish corrective surgery for these displacements

If the objective of disc repair is to return the disc to normal anatomy or as near as normal as possible, then the best time to do a disc repair would be before the anatomy has undergone any permanent deformation. Using Wilkes' classification for internal derangements,[28] it would appear that disc repair would be best performed in stage II and very early stage III internal derangements, in which there is clicking, pain and intermittent locking but slight if any changes of disc anatomy. This is the same stage at which non-surgical therapy has a good chance of being successful. Wilkes did an eight-year follow-up on 211 joints and found a 96.9% success rate in those cases in which disc repair was utilized.[22] He also found that disc repair was better than discectomy in the early stage cases (i.e., stage II and stage III).[22]

Unfortunately, the articles on disc repair that have been published are anything but uniform in many aspects. Many different procedures were utilized in trying to reposition the disc. Many other procedures were combined with a disc repair procedure, including condyloplasty or eminoplasty or both. There was no staging of internal derangements pre-operatively so in many instances stage IV and stage V cases were attempted to be corrected with disc repositioning procedures. Often the disc was re-contoured to try to return it to its original pre-displacement shape. The criteria for success were different in each article and, in fact, in several articles it was difficult to determine the overall success rate for disc repositioning procedures. Even more critical was the pre-operative selection of patients. Not only was the degree of displacement not identified, but also the degree of muscle dysfunction problems and other complicating factors was different for each group. Finally, post-operative management strategies of these patients were different in many of these articles. Modalities such as physical therapy, occlusal appliance therapy, orthodontics, orthognathic surgery, occlusal rehabilitation were or were not used, depending on the surgeon's philosophy. For these various reasons the treatment outcomes were very difficult to analyze and certainly impossible to combine together to reach any consensus or conclusions.

Six papers were reviewed which had at least six months follow-up and had repositioning of the disc as the only procedure accomplished. Marciani and Ziegler followed 10 patients over 35.5 months and found a 90% success rate, but unfortunately had no staging of the pre-operative disease.[29] Bronstein followed 17 patients (21 joints) over a one year time frame and found a 95% success rate.[30] The cases were stage II through V, and the only failure was a stage V patient. Dolwick and Sanders followed a series of patients for 18 months that had stage II and stage III disease pre-operatively and found an 85% improvement in function and pain reduction.[31] A 5.8 year follow-up on stage II-IV pre-operative disease had only a 62.5% success rate as reported by Politis et al.[32] In another study, that did not stage pre-operative disease and had a 6-24 month follow-up, a 90% success rate was reported.[33] Montgomery et al. followed 51 patients from 6 to 72 months with clinical examinations, questionnaires, and post-surgical joint imaging.[34] On the self-report, 95% of the patients reported improvement but 69% continued to have some residual pain. Of the patients treated with disc repositioning surgery, 54% were pre-operative stage III to stage V displacements.

In seven other articles not only disc repositioning surgery is described but also a form of bone recontouring as part of the procedure. McCarty and Farrar followed 327 joints from 6 to 27 months after disc repair surgery and a condyloplasty on the posterior aspect of the condyle and found a 94% success rate.[5] Unfortunately they did not describe any pre-operative staging. Mercuri et al. followed a small number of patients for over six months that had a disc repair procedure plus eminectomy and condyloplasty and found a 91.3% success rate, again with no pre-operative staging of the internal derangements.[35] Hall followed 20 temporomandibular joints with stage II to III pre-operative disease for 18.1 months and found, by doing only a superior lamina repair, that all patients improved.[36] Dolwick and Sanders accomplished a bone reduction procedure along with the disc repair on stage II and III patients and found a 90% success rate over 36 months.[31] A disco-condylar plication in which the disc is tied to the lateral pole of the condyle, had a 97% success rate over 1 to 2 years but with no pre-operative staging.[37] Kerstens et al. found 100% success by doing some type of arthroplasty to increase joint space along with a disc repair procedure on stage II patients and 81% success on stage III patients over 19.7 months.[38] Again with no report of pre-operative staging, 152 patients were followed for an average of eight years in which disc repair procedure was combined with some type of arthroplasty to increase joint space and a 90% success rate was found.[39]

Five papers reported on post-surgical imaging in order to determine the final position of the disc following disc repositioning surgery. Bronstein attempted arthrograms one year following the surgical procedure.[30] He found that four of 17 arthrograms were normal and four could not be accomplished. A post-operative arthrogram was found to be a very difficult procedure because of adhesions formed following the surgical repair of the disc. Zetz and Ash did post-operative magnetic resonance evaluations on 31 disc repair procedures

and found that 26 discs were in a normal position.[33] Unfortunately, there was
no clinical correlation as to post-operative disc position and rate of success.
The authors felt that the double layer closure of both the inferior and superior
lamina of the retrodiscal tissue was essential to hold the disc in the proper
position. Conway et al. found that the post-operative disc position correlated
with the clinical results and that the success of their particular patients was
technique sensitive.[40] In this magnetic resonance imaging study they compared
their successful surgical procedures against a series of patients that were
referred to them for post-operative magnetic resonance images after failure of
a surgical procedure. Thirty out of 35 surgically repositioned discs were found
to have returned to their pre-operative position on magnetic resonance imaging
according to Montgomery et al.[34] Of these patients, 68% continued to have
symptoms. A magnetic resonance imaging study on 46 patients 30 years after
initial evaluation found that the degree of deformity of the disc related to the
degree of displacement.[41] As long as the disc achieves an anterior superior
position on top of the condyle on opening, the disc will have a normal
bi-concave appearance. However, the configuration of the disc will deviate as
soon as the disc becomes permanently displaced.

Conclusions

As with all surgical procedures, patient selection is most important. Disc repair,
accomplished in early stages of reducing disc displacement, appears to be a
variable procedure in preventing further damage to the disc and other temporomandibular joint soft tissues. Once the disc becomes non-reducing, permanent
deformation occurs in all soft tissues. Magnetic resonance imaging is the best
procedure for post-operative evaluation of disc repair as long as metal is not
used as part of the repair technique. Surgical repair of the disc is very sensitive
with regard to the long-term success in relation to the technique used and the
skill of the surgeon. The future of disc repair surgery will rely on improving
the techniques in order to improve the stability of the disc to the condyle.
Long-term controlled studies on disc repair patients are needed to clear the air
on the success of this procedure. Can this procedure improve the natural course
of the disease? Can the number of facial deformities caused by temporomandibular joint osteoarthrosis be decreased by early disc repair? Only time
will tell!

References

1 Annandale T. On displacement of the interarticular cartilage of the lower jaw and its treatment by
   operation. Lancet 1887; 1:411
2 Behan RJ. Loose cartilage in the temporomandibular joint. Ann Surg 1918; 67:536
3 Norgaard F. Artrografi af kaebeldeddet: Preliminary report. Acta Radiol 1944; 25:679

4 Wilkes CH. Arthrography of the temporomandibular joint in patients with TMJ pain dysfunction syndrome. Minn Med 1978; 61:645
5 McCarty WL, Farrar WB. Surgery for internal derangement of the temporomandibular joint. J Prosthet Dent 1979; 42;191
6 Williams PL, Warwick R. Gray's anatomy. Edinburgh: Churchill Livingstone, 1980
7 Osborn JW. The disc of the human temporomandibular joint: design, function and failure. J Oral Rehabil 1985; 12:279
8 Rees LA. The structure and function of the temporomandibular joint. Br Dent J 1954; 96:125
9 Scapino RP. Histopathology associated with malposition of the human temporomandibular joint disc. Oral Surg Oral Med Oral Pathol 1983; 55:382
10 Griffin CJ, Hawthorn R, Harris R. Anatomy and histology of the human temporomandibular joint. Monogr Oral Sci 1975; 4:1
11 Griffin CJ, Sharpe CJ. Distribution of elastic tissue in the temporomandibular meniscus especially in respect to "compression" areas. Aust Dent J 1962; 7:72
12 Wilkes CH. Structural and functional alterations of the temporomandibular joint. Northw Dent 1978; 57:287
13 Boering G. Anatomical and physiological considerations regarding the temporomandibular joint. Int Dent J 1979; 29:245
14 Kurita K, Westesson PL, Sternby NH, et al. Histologic features of the temporomandibular joint disk and posterior disk attachment: Comparison of symptom-free persons with normally positioned disks and patients with internal derangement. Oral Surg Med Oral Pathol 1989; 67:635
15 Heffez LB, Jordan SL, Crawford GL. Geometric considerations of disk repositioning procedures. J Craniomandibular Pract 1993; 11:102
16 Westesson PL, Bronstein SL, Liedberg J. Internal derangement of the temporomandibular joint: morphologic description with correlation to joint function. Oral Surg Oral Med Oral Pathol 1985; 59:323
17 Luder HU. Articular degeneration and remodeling in human temporomandibular joints with normal and abnormal disc position. J Orofacial Pain 1993; 7:391
18 Isacsson G, Isberg A, Johansson AS, Larsson O. Internal derangement of the temporomandibular joint: radiographic and histologic changes associated with severe pain. J Oral Maxillofac Surg 1986; 44:771
19 Chase DC, McCoy JM. Histologic staging on internal derangement of the temporomandibular joint. Oral Maxillofac Surg Clin North Am 1989; 2:249
20 Hall MB, Brown RW, Baughman RA. Histologic appearance of the bilaminar zone in internal derangement of the temporomandibular joint. Oral Surg Oral Med Oral Path 1984; 58:375
21 Westesson PL, Lundh H. Arthrographic and clinical characteristics on patients with disk displacement who progressed to closed lock during a 6 month period. Oral Surg Oral Med Oral Pathol 1989; 67:654
22 Wilkes CH. Surgical treatment of internal derangements of the temporomandibular joint. Arch Otolaryngol Head Neck Surg 1991; 117:64
23 Hall MB, Baughman R, Ruskin J, Thompson DA. Healing following meniscoplasty eminectomy, and high condylectomy in the monkey temporomandibular joint. J Oral Maxillofac Surg 1986; 44:177
24 Eppley BL, Kalenderian E, Winkelmann T, Delfino JJ. Surgical repair on defects in the rabbit temporomandibular joint disc: a comparison of various techniques. J Oral Maxillofac Surg 1989; 47:587
25 McDonald F. The condyle disk as a controlling factor in the form of the condylar head. J Craniomandib Disord Facial Oral Pain 1989; 3:83
26 Bosanquet AG, Ishmaru JI, Goss AN. The effect of experimental disc perforation in sheep temporomandibular joints. Int J Oral Maxillofac Surg 1991; 20:177
27 Ali AM, Sharawy M, O'Dell NL, Al-Behery G. Morphological alterations in the elastic fibers of the rabbit craniomandibular joint following experimentally induced anterior disk displacement. Acta Anat 1993; 147:159
28 Wilkes CH. Internal derangements of the temporomandibular joint. Arch Otolaryngol Head Neck Surg 1989; 115:469
29 Marciani R, Ziegler R. Temporomandibular joint surgery: a review of fifty-one operations. Oral Surg Oral Med Oral Pathol 1983; 56:472
30 Bronstein SL. Post-surgical TMJ arthrography. J Craniomandibular Pract 1984; 2:165

31 Dolwick MF, Sanders B. TMJ internal derangement and arthrosis: surgical atlas. St Louis: Mosby, 1985; 202

32 Politis C, Stoelinga PJW, Gerritsen GW, Heyboer A. Long-term results of surgical intervention on the temporomandibular joint. J Craniomandibular Pract 1989; 7:319

33 Zetz M, Ash D. Double-layer closure for temporomandibular joint discoplasty. J Oral Maxillofac Surg 1989; 47:427

34 Montgomery MT, Gordon SM, VanSickels JE, Harms SE. Changes in signs and symptoms following temporomandibular joint disc repositioning surgery. J Oral Maxillofac Surg 1992; 50:320

35 Mercuri L, Campbell R, Shamaskin R. Intra-articular meniscal dysfunction surgery. Oral Surg Oral Med Oral Pathol 1982; 54:613

36 Hall MB. Meniscoplasty of the displaced temporomandibular joint meniscus without violating the inferior joint space. J Oral Maxillofac Surg 1984; 42:788

37 Weinberg S, Cousens G. Meniscocondylar plication: a modified operation for surgical repositioning of the ectopic temporomandibular joint meniscus. Oral Surg Oral Med Oral Pathol 1987; 63:393

38 Kerstens HCJ, Tuinzing DB, van der Kwast WAM. Eminectomy and discoplasty for correction of the displaced temporomandibular joint disc. J Oral Maxillofac Surg 1989; 47:150

39 Dolwick MF, Nitzan DW. TMJ disk surgery: an 8 year follow-up evaluation. Fortschr Kiefer Gesichts Chir 1990; 35:162

40 Conway WF, Hayes CW, Campbell RL, Laskin DM, Swanson KS. Temporomandibular joint after meniscoplasty: appearance at MR Imaging. Radiology 1991; 180:749

41 de Leeuw R, Boering G, Stegenga B, de Bont LGM. Temporomandibular joint articular disk position and configuration 30 years after diagnosis of internal derangement: a magnetic resonance imaging study. In: de Leeuw R. A thirty-year follow-up study of non-surgically treated temporomandibular joint osteoarthrosis and internal derangement. Thesis, University of Groningen, The Netherlands, 1994

Post-operative care
and treatment failure

Management of Temporomandibular
Joint Degenerative Diseases
ed. by B. Stegenga & L.G.M. de Bont
© 1996 Birkhäuser Verlag Basel/Switzerland

Rehabilitation of the temporomandibular joint through the application of motion

William L. McCarty Jr.

Oral and Maxillofacial Surgery, Baptist Medical Center, Montgomery, Alabama 36198, USA

Summary: This chapter presents a method of joint rehabilitation using the principles of active motion, continuous passive motion, and reduction of joint loading. The physiologically sound principles of joint mobilization are used both as post-surgical rehabilitation and as definitive therapy. When used as non-surgical therapy, the benefits appear to be the result of a reversal, lessening, or favorable adaptive response to chemical and mechanical alterations.

Introduction

Substantial gains in knowledge of temporomandibular joint anatomy, physiology, disease and dysfunction have been made over the last 20 years. These gains have primarily been secondary to observation at the time of surgery, joint imaging, arthroscopic observations, and outcomes and anatomical studies on both a macroscopic and microscopic level.[1-19] Many treatment options have been proposed for this complex joint. One area which received little attention on a clinical level has been the physiological effects of motion on arthropathies. This study will focus on rehabilitation through application of motion to improve dysfunctional components, thus reducing pain. The initial premise for the rehabilitation method is based on the following observations:

- The majority of patients with symptomatic arthropathies have a restricted range of motion, and the motion most often affected is translation.
- Review of approximately 75 reconstructive arthroplasty patients of at least 10 years duration showed a definite relationship between long-term success and range of motion. It was evident that patients with the ability to translate were more successful, in spite of the fact that the vast majority of those patients still had marked intra-articular pathology.
- Among the general population of patients, an abundance of joint pathology is present; yet, a distinct lack of significant symptoms is referable to the temporomandibular joint. These patients, despite pathological changes (both clinically and radiographically), have a good range of motion and no significant dysfunction. This group is very similar to the above-mentioned surgery patients. No significant symptoms were found 10 years after surgery, range of motion was good, and joints were pathologic.

These observations lead to the conclusion that the degree of intra-articular pathology is not parallel to the degree of symptoms, and that the range of motion appears to be a significant variable relative to symptoms. Long-term unresolved dysfunction leads to further pathological changes, both intra- and extra-articular. Although there are exceptions, if pathological changes are not accompanied by significant dysfunction in terms of decreased range of motion, symptoms appear to be relatively minor and cyclic. The conclusions based upon these observations would lead one to think that a poor correlation exists between pathology and pain, but a good correlation between pathology accompanied by dysfunction and pain. The goal of the rehabilitation method presented in this chapter is to reduce symptoms by reducing the dysfunctional component (i.e., restricted range of motion) and allowing for a favorable adaptive response of pathology.

Principal movements of the temporomandibular joint

The two principal motions of the temporomandibular joint are rotation and translation. During normal function, they work together. Although there are normal variations, the first movement in a healthy joint is the condyle rotating to approximately 25 mm of interincisal opening. This is followed by a translatory motion of the condyle to a full range of opening. Normal is considered to be 40-50 mm. In a normal joint, an approximate 4:1 ratio exists between maximum opening and maximum translation, as measured by lateral excursions to the opposite side or by protrusion.[20] If the mouth can open 40 mm, the expected lateral motion should be 10 mm. This ratio is clinically important, as it will assist in determining if the restricted range of motion is primarily intra- or extra-articular. Using only maximum interincisal opening as the parameter of function is incomplete and misleading. Interincisal opening can be taken as a general measurement of extra-articular function, and the ability to translate as that of intra-articular function, with the 4:1 ratio combining the two measurements. If the ability to translate is the primary measurement of intra-articular function, then translation becomes the most important movement relative to intra-articular disorders. However, this does not mean that rotation is not important. Both are important to normal function. Many conditions affect the temporomandibular joint where the ability to rotate is unaffected, but the ability to translate is reduced. This is especially true following intra-articular procedures, trauma, protracted periods of total or partial immobilization, as well as pain and dysfunction secondary to internal derangements and degenerative diseases. If the primary rehabilitative effort is to achieve normal interincisal opening, this can most often be achieved, but the ability to translate may remain limited and may never be regained, resulting in a progressively dysfunctional and painful joint. On the other hand, if translation is the primary goal of rehabilitation, then rotation/interincisal opening will occur as a normal course of events, unless there is an ongoing extra-articular reason for restriction. In general, if a joint can translate it can rotate. But if it rotates, it will not necessarily translate.

Restrictions in motion secondary to altered joint mechanics and pathology do not have a single cause. Internal derangement is generally a progressive disorder, beginning with reducing disc displacements of varying degrees. Late- and mid-reductions are commonly associated with transient locking. Permanent disc displacement is characterized by an acute phase, commonly termed "closed-lock", with a transition to the chronic phase over a variable period of time. Degenerative bone changes have been thought to occur secondary to the advanced stages of internal derangement. However, recent studies have shown that these changes are significantly present, even during stages with a reducing disc.[21] Reasons for restriction of motion will vary, depending upon the stage of joint pathology and impairment of joint mechanics. Restriction of motion can be actual, as a result of mechanical events, secondary to pain, or in combination. During the early stages of internal derangement, the majority of restriction is probably secondary to pain or hypertrophy of the posterior band in some cases. Restriction of motion or partial immobilization may contribute to chemical changes within the joint, such as an alteration of synovial fluid with resultant changes of the frictional quality of the bearing surfaces contributing to or hastening the osteoarthrotic process. Restriction during the 'middle stages' of internal derangement (characterized by transient and permanent locking) are secondary to mechanical blocking of the disc, as well as alterations of the gliding surfaces of hard and soft tissue components and pain. With the later stages (i.e., permanent disc displacement and residual osteoarthrosis) restriction of motion is most probably secondary to the pathological and mechanical events which have led to this stage, such as advanced degree of displacement with distortion, synovitis, adhesions, pain, and degenerative changes. Capsular fibrosis, seen commonly in joints with osteoarthrosis, may further contribute to restriction of motion. Capsular tightness may also cause a decrease in fluid nutrients entering the joint, as well as decreasing the ability for waste products to be removed. This further contributes to the cycle of joint stiffness, decreased gliding, and pain. It would appear that many of these mechanical and chemical alterations have an origin in some degree of immobility, or that lack of normal motion is a contributor.

Continuous passive motion

Review

Continuous passive motion is now a widely accepted modality in orthopedic rehabilitation. This is especially true during the early phases of post-operative management of knees, hips, shoulders, hands, fingers, ankles, and toes. As long as safe limits of tissue healing are observed, early motion with controlled forces act on collagen tissues by maintaining nutrition through improved fluid dynamics. This decreases the effects of disuse and retarding capsular contracture and joint stiffness.

Conceptually, Salter et al. began performing several experimental animal studies on the effects of continuous passive motion on soft tissue healing, bone and cartilage healing, edema, haemarthrosis, and joint function.[22] Controversy between rest versus motion has long been debated. Unfortunately, the trends that developed were seldom based upon sound scientific research principles. As the ill-effects of immobilization began to be documented, it became apparent that in many cases early motion was necessary to ultimately restore optimal functional use of the anatomy. Since Salter and co-workers published their landmark study in 1980, a number of subsequent studies have been published to substantiate their findings as well as extend our knowledge of joint and soft tissue healing principles.[23] As a result, continuous passive motion is now considered the rule rather than the exception in the management of certain orthopedic post-operative cases or manipulative procedures. Continuous passive motion is not meant to be a replacement for active exercise or for any other aspect of a patient's normal rehabilitation. Instead, it augments the patient's rehabilitation regimen by facilitating a speedier and more physiologically sound recovery. Continuous passive motion is probably as much of a philosophy as it is a modality.

Immobilization, whether prescribed as a form of treatment or as a pathological condition, has been recognized clinically in humans and experimentally in animals as having detrimental effects on bone and soft tissue homeostasis. Changes include mechanical, histological and biomechanical alterations.[23] Immobilization creates excessive fatty fibrous connective tissue which forms mature scars and creates intra-articular adhesions. This fatty fibrous connective tissue will encroach upon the joint cleft, envelop ligaments, and become confluent with unopposed articular surfaces, which may eventually obliterate the joint cavity.[23,24] Restricted range of motion due to capsular fibrosis creates a distinct reduction in the blood supply to the joint capsule. Capsular tightness causes improper loading of articular cartilage. A fibrous capsule does not allow normal arthrokinematic movements to occur. Capsular tightness will cause certain areas of the articular cartilage to receive higher impact loads, possibly leading to fatigue and degenerative changes.[25] Prolonged immobilization causes a gradual resorption of the articular cartilage with further fibrofatty tissue encroachment. Events then may proceed to include abutment against the subchondral bone and in some instances communication with the bone marrow. Immobilization provides for the stationary position needed for abnormal collagen fiber cross-link formation resulting in adhesions.[26,27]

Motion inhibits contracture formation by stimulating synthesis of glycosaminoglycans, which maintains lubrication and critical fiber distance by directing an orderly deposition of new collagen fibers. Studies have shown that limited motion of 3-5 mm is sufficient to prevent the formation of adhesions between repaired tendons and the digital sheath.[27]

Fluid dynamics are also affected by immobilization and, if compromised, will lead to further degeneration. Due to immobilization, the synovial membrane gradually adheres to the cartilage and over time the membrane obliterates the joint and prevents joint nutrition.[28] Without full range of motion, synovial fluid will mix inadequately. Through diminished fluid dynamics, waste products of metabolism will accumulate on the cartilage surfaces, causing cartilage cell dystrophy. When tissue injury occurs, prostaglandins, bradykinin, histamine, serotonin, leukotrienes, thromboxanes, and platelet activating factors are released. These substances cause congestion in the capillary bed and extravasation of fluid into the extravascular space.[29] Along with stress-induced release of epinephrine and norepinephrine, these mediators will constrict precapillary arterioles thus restricting fluid dynamics to the interstitial spaces.[30] Lymph channels are highways to clear congestion during the inflammatory process. These lymph vessels rely upon the action of skeletal muscles and motion to pump lymphatic fluid through the system. Mobility dysfunction, whether acute or chronic, will inhibit lymphatic clearing. An inflammation-edema cycle can easily develop and will further contribute to degenerative joint breakdown, adhesion formation, capsular fibrosis, and other responses.[31] When inflammation exceeds its useful function, harmful effects occur such as proliferative scar tissue formation and tissue destruction. As efforts are introduced to increase joint mobility, fluid dynamics begin to improve.

A third way that continuous passive motion exerts a positive effect to a joint is through normalized mechanoreceptor activity. All synovial joints of the body are provided with four varieties of receptor nerve endings. Types I, II and III are static or dynamic articular mechanoreceptors. Activation of these mechanoreceptors contribute to the perceptual experiences of postural sensation and kinesthesia. Type IV receptors are nociceptors that are normally inactive but become active when abnormally high tensions develop in the articular tissues. Capsular fibrosis affecting mechanoreceptor activity contributes to improper joint proprioceptive feedback and jaw muscle activity. Capsular distention occurring with joint effusion will also alter mechanoreceptor activity. High tensions in articular tissue may develop due to excessive adhesion formation or alterations in fluid dynamics. Type IV mechanoreceptors are also activated when exposed to high concentrations of irritant chemical substances during inflammation. Motion stimulates types I, II and III mechanoreceptor activity, thereby exerting reciprocally coordinated reflexogenic influences on muscle tone and on the excitability of stretch reflexes in all striated muscles. Afferent discharges form these mechanoreceptors converge on inhibitory interneurons, segmentally and intersegmentally, thus modulating the centripetal flow of type IV nociceptor afferent activity. The intensity of type IV irritation coupled with the frequency of ongoing afferent discharges from types I, II and III mechanoreceptors will determine the degree of arthralgia. Deliberate stimulation of types I, II and III mechanoreceptors by an intervention such as motion will damp down the transmission of type IV activity through the synapses in the basal spinal nucleus and impede the flow up into the brain to evoke the experience of pain.[25,32]

Continuous passive motion device

In the 1980s, because of frustration with multiple surgery patients, the notion of a rehabilitative method using the principles of active and passive motion was conceived primarily as a result of the obvious relationship between restricted range of motion and pain, the importance of translation, and a clinical need for post-operative patients to rapidly return to a more normal range of motion. The importance of joint mobilization has been amplified by our knowledge of the physiological effect of continuous passive motion.

Since the first prototype of the current continuous passive motion device, which was used in 1987, four others have been developed. Changes in prototype development have progressed along the lines of safety, patient comfort and acceptance, device size, means for tooth engagement, patient set-up, simplicity of administration, and protocols for therapy. The same principles have applied throughout, i.e., a continuous passive motion device operating in a horizontal plane, thereby promoting the ability of the patient to translate.

Rehabilitation

Principles

Rehabilitation uses the principles of active and passive motion and decreased joint loading. The chief function of rehabilitation is confined to the direct effects on intra-articular structures. Passive motion is achieved with the application of the continuous passive motion device, while active motion is performed by the patient. The device provides the benefits of continuous passive motion, joint mobilization, and also assists the patient in the proper performance of active motion. Decreased joint loading is achieved by strict adherence to diet modification and the use of an occlusal appliance.

The continuous passive motion device is a hand held, motorized unit that imparts translatory motion to the joints by means of a moveable lower plate, which functions in a horizontal plane. The system uses incrementally graded cams to gradually increase the range of motion at a variable speed. Cam increases are controlled by the therapist, and speed is selected by the patient. Strict therapy protocols are difficult to determine, as each patient must be considered on an individual basis. Treatment protocols have been worked out over the past several years, judging individual patient response and being guided by the fact that therapy has to be reasonable if compliance is expected. A useful treatment protocol consists of four sessions daily, spaced evenly, for 2-10 minutes each session. Incorporation of motion is incremental and progressively graded, both in terms of degree of motion and length of time. Little emphasis is place on increasing interincisal opening, except by having the patient gently stretch and hold it for a few seconds. Attempts to affect maximum interincisal opening by forced movement appears to be detrimental to soft tissues, which in the majority of cases of chronic hypomobility has undergone adaptive shortening. The immediate goal post-operatively is to achieve intra-articular translation. Passive motion will assist the proper development of active motion by helping to reduce extra-articular soft tissue swelling and irritability. Post-operative cases must be viewed as a race against time, as the process of adhesion formation will occur immediately. If extra-articular soft tissue is traumatized by sudden forced movements, then muscle pain will greatly restrict motion. The length of time required for the use of the device varies, depending upon the pathological condition of the joint, as well as patient compliance. The average time required for use of the device is approximately two to four weeks.

Clinical application: post-operative patients

Material and methods
The rehabilitation method has been used in a multicenter clinical setting with post-operative patients, divided into three categories, i.e., initial or first time open joint surgery, patients who have had one or more previous open joint procedures, and total joint replacement.

The initial surgery patients involved a total of 60 joints (30 joints treated with the described rehabilitation method, and 30 joints as controls). Data were taken from patients' files on a consecutive basis. Pathological conditions were distributed evenly between both groups, the majority having permanent disc displacement with some degree of degenerative changes. There were a total of 14 perforations, all occurring within the retrodiscal tissue. Patients in both groups had high pain levels, which were directly attributable to intra-articular pathology and dysfunction. All patients had complete work-ups including tomograms and arthrograms. Patients in both groups had an average duration of symptoms of three years with an average age of 35; 95% were female. There were two reconstructive arthroplasties, one arthroplasty with a Christianson implant, and the remainder were discectomies without an implant of any type. In both groups rehabilitation was started the day following surgery, and the majority of patients were seen for five consecutive working days for physical therapy consisting of application of ice, ultrasound and active translatory exercises. The group using the continuous passive motion device typically started with a 0.5 mm cam and gradually progressed up to 4 and 5 mm cams. Average length of time to use the device was approximately two weeks. Average follow-up time was 11 months.

Regarding multiple surgery patients, again, the only difference between the study and control groups (20 patients each) was the addition of the continuous passive motion device. The 20 patients representing the continuous passive motion group had a total of 28 previous surgeries, while the control group had 22. All patients in both groups had marked degenerative changes. There were 24 cases of severe fibrous ankylosis and eight cases of bony ankylosis.

Pathology was fairly evenly distributed between the two groups. Pre-operative evaluation was identical to that of the initial surgery group, with the exception of arthrography. Post-operative protocols were identical to the initial surgery group, the main difference being that this group was much more difficult, and the post-operative course was more protracted. Average use of the device was approximately one month. Average follow-up was eight months.

In the total joint replacement group, the continuous passive motion device was used on 18 patients with 18 used for control. All patients had bilateral total joint replacements using Viteck, Techmedica and Osteomed prostheses. On five patients, the device was instituted immediately after surgery.

Results
Objective results for the initial surgery patients are listed in table 1, and those for multiple surgery patients in table 2. In the total joint replacement groups, on four of the patients the device was used anywhere from three months to one year post-operatively. In those four instances, there was no positive effect. When the device was used immediately following surgery, lateral range of motion more than doubled that of the control group.

In the initial surgery group, when comparing the continuous passive motion and control groups, no statistical differences were measured in range of motion prior to surgery. After surgery, however, the continuous passive motion group had significantly ($p < .01$) greater ranges of motion than did the control group. Statistical tests for homogenicity were also performed to assess the subjective responses as reported by the patients. For the initial surgery patients, 28 patients in the continuous passive motion group and 27 patients in the control group had excellent or good results. Patients in the continuous passive motion group reported significantly ($p < .01$) more excellent subjective responses to treatment than did the control group.

Table 1. Ranges of motion (mm) for initial surgery patients

Range of motion	Before surgery		After surgery and rehabilitation	
	Mean	SD*	Mean	SD*
*CPM-group***				
Max. opening	36.6	6.9	43.3	3.9
Lateral				
to opposite side	6.1	1.6	9.7	1.1
to affected side	7.5	1.9	10.5	1.4
Control group				
Max. opening	36.7	4.7	40.5	3.1
Lateral				
to opposite side	7.1	1.8	8.3	1.3
to affected side	8.5	1.7	9.6	1.1

* SD = standard deviation
** CPM = continuous passive motion

Table 2. Ranges of motion (mm) for multiple surgery patients

Range of motion	Before surgery		After surgery and rehabilitation	
	Mean	SD*	Mean	SD*
*CPM-group***				
Max. opening	26.8	8.0	38.6	3.7
Lateral				
to opposite side	3.4	1.9	7.4	2.0
to affected side	5.4	2.6	8.5	2.4
Control group				
Max. opening	26.1	6.1	34.8	5.0
Lateral				
to opposite side	3.6	1.5	5.5	1.2
to affected side	6.6	1.4	7.8	1.2

* SD = standard deviation
** CPM = continuous passive motion

Statistical paired comparisons were also performed for the multiple surgery groups. Both groups had significantly ($p < .01$) greater ranges of motion after surgery than before surgery. The differences between the continuous passive motion and the control group, however, were not as favorable in the multiple surgery patients as they were for the initial surgery patients. Only the range of motion for "lateral to opposite side" showed a significant ($p > .01$) increase for the continuous passive motion group as compared with the control group. Subjective responses from the multiple surgery patients were also analyzed. No significant differences in reported responses existed between the continuous passive motion and control groups. In both groups, eight patients reported an excellent or good result.

Discussion
The surgical outcomes of the initial surgery group reflected favorably in both the continuous passive motion and the control groups. However, both the objective and subjective parameters showed significant improvement in the continuous passive motion group. This group also gained sufficient motion more quickly, probably due to the benefits of continuous passive motion as discussed previously and also by aiding in performance and compliance of active exercises. For the most part, the control group tended to have a lot of frustration and difficulty in performance of active exercises. Frustration was also associated with the administration of post-operative therapy. Addition of the device was favorable relative to time and ease of post-operative management.

The multiple surgery patient group was disappointing in symptom reduction in both groups. Addition of the continuous passive motion device, however, showed a significant increase in translation to the opposite side over the group where the device was not used. The reasons for improvement are probably the same as with the initial surgery group. Multiple surgery patients have increased intra-articular pathology in addition to adaptive shortening of masticatory muscles and soft tissues. Post-operatively, multiple surgery patients are much more difficult to manage. The majority of these patients have higher pain levels. It would be expected over a longitudinal period that if these patients can maintain or improve their range of motion, symptoms should likewise improve. It is an observation that unless a patient can regain and maintain a lateral excursion to the opposite side of 7 or 8 mm within a month after surgery, the outlook is guarded. One lesson to be learned is that the first surgery has the best chance and if a relative normal range of motion has not been regained quickly, the chances of ongoing pain or repeat surgery increases.

The continuous passive motion device is effective in increasing mobility with total joint replacement if therapy is instituted immediately after surgery. Even though the degree of lateral motion is not great, it is significant in the effect of reducing adhesions between the surfaces of the prosthesis. With the loss of the lateral pterygoid muscles, any translatory motion would have to be supplied by the temporalis and deep portion of the masseter muscle with perhaps some help from the digastric.

Adhesion formation will occur rapidly following any type of open joint procedure. The post-operative goal is the creation of a pseudo-arthrosis with organized scar tissue as opposed to disorganized scar tissue attaching to the bearing surfaces resulting in bone softening, ankylosis and resorptive remodeling. This will occur if the range of motion, and especially the ability to translate, is not returned quickly after surgery. A discectomy with no implant is an excellent surgical procedure where indicated, but must be followed by a quick return of motion if success is to be achieved.

Clinical application: definitive and adjunctive therapy

The most interesting application of the rehabilitation and the one with perhaps the most significant clinical implication is its use as definitive or adjunctive therapy. It was observed that patients undergoing unilateral surgery, but with some degree of pain on the opposite side, had a decrease in symptoms on that side following post-operative rehabilitation with the continuous passive motion device. It was assumed that this was probably a result of the post-operative rehabilitation. As a result of this observation, the application of motion to painful arthropathies has been used as definitive or adjunctive therapy.

Material and methods

The term adjunctive therapy applies because in all instances, reduction of joint loading was accomplished through strict diet modification and in some instances an occlusal appliance of 2 mm thickness was used, not to achieve occlusal change, but to help prevent excessive loading.

All 26 patients had symptoms referable to articular temporomandibular disorders. All but three patients had previous unsuccessful treatment by some

Table 3. Ranges of motion (mm) for total joint replacements

Range of motion	Before surgery Mean	After surgery and rehabilitation Mean
*CPM-group**		
Max. opening	17	32
Lateral		
to opposite side	1	5
to affected side	2	5
Control group		
Max. opening	17	29
Lateral		
to opposite side	1	2
to affected side	2	2

* CPM= continuous passive motion

form of occlusal modification. Patients in this category were selected primarily because of proximity and a "willingness for experimentation". Corrected serial tomograms and arthrography were used to make a specific diagnosis.

Results

Results of this therapy are summarized in Table 4. The results were favorable in producing range of motion improvements. Paired comparisons before and after treatment showed significant ($p < 0.01$) improvements in all three range of motion measures. However, subjective responses reported during this treatment were not homogeneous with responses reported by patients who were surgically treated. A high percentage (61.5%) of the definitive-adjunctive group reported excellent results, yet 26.9% subjectively reported this treatment had failed. No one was worse.

Discussion

It would appear that the application of motion to painful joints is effective in relief of symptoms. Specific conclusions as to why this occurs are debatable. In order to answer this question properly, a full understanding of reasons for arthralgia would have to exist. At the present time, however, there appears to be no concrete answer. Possibilities would include mechanical nerve compression secondary to disc displacement, neurogenic inflammation secondary to intra-articular chemical change and synovitis, adhesions, and osteoarthrosis. Even though arthrotic change may occur independently of an internal derangement, these bone changes are most often associated with significant disc displacements, in addition to alterations in chemical and/or fluid dynamics which cause inflammation and adhesions.

An answer as to why the application of motion can resolve symptoms secondary to pathology and dysfunction have been discussed in previous sections of this chapter. One other possibility exists, and this is mainly specu-

Table 4. Ranges of motion (mm) and patient profile for definitive/adjunctive treatment

Range of motion	Before surgery		After surgery and rehabilitation	
	Mean	SD*	Mean	SD*
Max. opening	35.1	6.3	40.4	4.4
Lateral				
to opposite side	6.7	1.3	9.3	1.3
to affected side	9.1	1.4	10.3	0.8

Patient profile

Category	Number of joints
Reducing disc displacement	6
Permanent disc displacement	15
Acute closed-lock	2
Previous surgery	3

* SD= standard deviation

lation. Changes in quality of the retrodiscal tissue have been observed histologically,[33,34] as well as in both open joint surgery and arthroscopic procedures.[35] The speculation is that if controlled motion or irritation is applied to a tissue surface, the result is a cellular change affecting the quality of the tissue. An analogy would be the development of a callous on a skin surface which is brought about by controlled irritation and results in protection from the irritant. Obviously the retrodiscal tissue is not composed of epidermis, but it is possible for a similar phenomenon to occur. Much like skin surfaces, if the application of the irritant is excessive, blisters and ulcerations occur. If the irritant, in this case motion, is controlled and graduated and excessive irritants are reduced by reduction of joint loading, then reorganization of the cellular make-up of the retrodiscal tissue is possible with resultant pain reduction. It is possible that this is the mechanism for pain reduction in three of the patients that had fairly normal ranges of motion and no radiographic evidence of advanced degenerative changes.

The two patients with acute closed-locks (table 4) derived no significant benefit from the rehabilitation. Subsequently, arthrocentesis was administered. One patient showed an improvement in range of motion and symptoms, despite the fact that disc position did not change. The three previous surgery patients were all successful and of several years duration with acute exacerbations of joint pain; reasons are unknown. As the range of motion was more normalized, the symptoms decreased. The six patients with reducing disc displacement had restricted ranges of motion despite the fact that reduction was verified with arthrography. Pain would appear to be the primary implicator as the reason for restricted motion.

Average length of time to use the continuous passive motion device on definitive patients was approximately two weeks. It would appear that if significant benefits were not gained within a two week period of time, this form of therapy would probably not be beneficial.

Use of the rehabilitation has not been used to date with post-arthroscopic cases. However, it would seem apparent that it would be beneficial. Even though arthroscopic procedures are not in general as traumatic as open joint surgery, there is soft tissue injury to the capsule and often some degree of haemarthrosis. The rehabilitation should obtund the effect of these sequelae, lessening adhesions and potentiate or maintain the mobility between the superior surface of the disc and the temporal component.

Summary and conclusions

It is apparent that there is no single cause for the production of symptoms in temporomandibular arthropathies. It appears rather that it is a cascading effect of both mechanical and chemical alterations. It is probable that one major common denominator in the production of symptoms would be secondary to the effects of restricted motion. As the effects of immobilization or hypomobility are known, it would be logical that beneficial effects could be derived from the application of motion. Possible reasons for these beneficial effects would include improved fluid dynamics through a pumping action and/or expansion of a fibrotic capsule, stimulation of mechanoreceptor or obtund pain, preventing or lessening the restrictive/painful effects of adhesions, and possibly aid in the formation of a pseudo-disc or, in some manner, alter the quality of the retrodiscal tissue which is subject to compression neuropathy.

Use of rehabilitation has been illustrated with two distinct categories, i.e. post-operative and definitive/adjunctive therapy. Post-operatively, the rehabilitation is beneficial in reducing intra-articular adhesions, thereby promoting a more normal range of motion and lessening chances for continuing pain or repeat surgery. With definitive/adjunctive therapy, the application of motion to painful joint disorders certainly appears to be beneficial with pain reduction occurring as a result of a variety of reasons, probably depending upon at what point that motion is applied in the progression of the disorder. It is possible that the application of motion could have a preventive effect by lessening the sum of the cascading effects of both mechanical and chemical alterations.

The described rehabilitation method is not intended to supplant any other logical and proven form of therapy for the treatment of temporomandibular arthropathies, but is presented as a potentiator of other forms of therapy. Further studies are obviously needed to fully assess this apparently novel but physiologically sound form of therapy.

References

1 Farrar WB. Characteristics of the condylar path in internal derangements of the temporomandibular joint. J Prosthet Dent 1978; 39:319
2 Boering G. Temporomandibular joint arthrosis: an analysis of 400 cases. Thesis, University of Groningen, The Netherlands, 1966
3 de Bont LGM, Boering G, Liem RSB, et al. Osteoarthrosis of the temporomandibular joint: a light microscopic and scanning electron microscopic study of the articular cartilage of the mandibular condyle. J Oral Maxillofac Surg 1985; 43:481
4 de Bont LGM, Liem RSB, Boering G. Ultrastructure of the articular cartilage of the mandibular condyle: ageing and degeneration. Oral Surg Oral Med Oral Pathol 1985; 60:631
5 Isacsson G, Isberg A. Tissue identification of the temporomandibular joint disk attachments and related vascularization. J Craniomandibular Pract 1985; 3:374
6 Isberg-Holm A. Temporomandibular joint clicking. Thesis, Karolinksa Institutet Stockholm, Sweden, 1980
7 Farrar WB, McCarty WL. Inferior joint space arthrography and characteristics of condylar paths in internal derangements with the temporomandibular joint. J Prosthet Dent 1979; 41:458
8 Katzberg RW, Dolwick MF, Holms CA, et al. Arthrography of the temporomandibular joint. AJR 1980; 134:995
9 Ohnishi M. Arthroscopy of the human temporomandibular joint. J Jpn Stomatol Soc 1975; 42:207
10 Murakami K, Hoshino K. Histological studies on the inner surfaces of the articular cavities of human temporomandibular joints with special reference to arthroscopic observations. Anat Anz 1985; 160:167
11 Holmlund A, Hellsing G. Arthroscopy of the temporomandibular joint. Int J Oral Maxillofac Surg 1985; 14:169
12 Saunders B, Boncristini R. Diagnostic and surgical arthroscopy of the temporomandibular joint. Clinical experience with 137 procedures over a 2-year period. J Craniomand Disorders Facial Oral Pain 1986; 1:202
13 McCain J, De la Rua H. Principles and practice of operative arthroscopy of the human temporomandibular joint. Oral Maxillofac Surg Clin North Am 1989; 1:135
14 Wilkes CH. Structural and functional alterations of the temporomandibular joint. Northwest Dent 1978; 57:287
15 Schellhas KP, Wilkes CH, Fritts HM, et al. Temporomandibular joint: MR imaging of internal derangements and post-operative changes. Am J Radiol 1988; 150:381
16 Nitzan DW, Dolwick MF, Martinez A. Temporomandibular joint arthrocentesis: a simplified treatment for severe limited mouth opening. J Oral Maxillofac Surg 1991; 49:1163
17 Kirk W. Morphological differences between superior and inferior disc surfaces in chronic internal derangements of the temporomandibular joint. J Oral Maxillofac Surg 1990; 48:455
18 Glineburg R, Laskin D, Blaustein D. The effect of immobilization on the primate temporomandibular joint. J Oral Maxillofac Surg 1982; 40:3
19 Eriksson L. Diagnosis and surgical treatment of internal derangement of the temporomandibular joint. Swed Dent J Suppl 25, 1985
20 Farrar WB, McCarty WL. A clinical outline of temporomandibular joint diagnosis and treatment. 7th ed. Montgomery: Normandie, 1982
21 Stegenga B. Temporomandibular joint osteoarthrosis and internal derangement. Diagnostic and therapeutic outcome assessment. Thesis, University of Groningen, The Netherlands, 1991
22 Salter RB, Simmonds DF, Malcolm BW, et al. The biological effects of continuous passive motion on the healing of full thickness defects in articular cartilage: an experimental investigation in the rabbit. J Bone Joint Surg (Am) 1980; 62:232
23 McCarthy MR, O'Donoghue PC, Yates CK, Yates-McCarthy JL. The clinical use of continuous passive motion in physical therapy. JOSPT 1992; 15:132
24 Poremba EP, Moffett BC. The effects of continuous passive motion on the temporomandibular joint after surgery. Oral Surg Oral Med Oral Pathol 1989; 67:490
25 Kraus SL. Management of the craniomandibular complex. In: Kraus SL (ed). Clinics in physical therapy: temporomandibular disorders. New York: Churchill Livingstone, 1988
26 Enneking WF, Horowitz H. The intra-articular effects of immobilization on the human knee. J Bone Joint Surg 1972; 54A:973

27 Gelberman RH. Influences of the protected passive mobilization interval on flexortendon healing. Clin Orthop Rel Res 1991; 264:189

28 Salter RB. The healing of articular tissues through continuous passive motion. Essence of the first ten years of experimental investigations. J Bone Joint Surg 1982; 64B:640

29 Rubin E, Farber JL. Pathology. Seranton: Lippencott, 1988

30 Guyton AC. Textbook of medical physiology. Philadelphia: Saunders, 1976

31 Mahan PE. The temporomandibular joint function and pathofunction. In: Solberg W, Clark GT (eds). Temporomandibular joint problems: biologic diagnosis and treatment. Chicago: Quintessence, 1980; 33

32 Wyke BD. The neurology of joints: a review of general principles. Clin Rheum Dis 1981; 7:223

33 Scapino RP. Histopathology associated with malposition of the human temporomandibular joint disc. Oral Surg 1983;55:382

34 Hall MB, Brown RW, Baughman RA. Histologic appearance of the bilaminar zone in internal derangement of the temporomandibular joint. Oral Surg Oral Med Oral Pathol 1984; 58:375

35 Blaustein D, Heffez I. Diagnostic arthroscopy of the temporomandibular joint. II. Arthroscopic findings of arthrographically diagnosed disk displacements. Oral Surg Oral Med Oral Pathol 1988; 65:135

This chapter is based on the article previously published in CRANIO: The Journal of Craniomandibular Practice 1993; 11(4):298-307. Reprinted with permission.

Management of Temporomandibular
Joint Degenerative Diseases
ed. by B. Stegenga & L.G.M. de Bont
© 1996 Birkhäuser Verlag Basel/Switzerland

Post-operative physical therapy of the temporomandibular joint

Pieter U. Dijkstra

*Department of Oral and Maxillofacial Surgery, Division of Physical Therapy, Department of
Rehabilitation, University Hospital Groningen, 9700 RB Groningen, The Netherlands*

Summary: The available physical therapy protocols after temporomandibular joint surgery are reviewed. In the immediate post-operative phase, physical therapy is provided primarily to reduce the
traumatizing effects of surgery. In later post-operative phases, treatment is aimed at mobilizing joints
and rehabilitating muscles. Eventually, the aim is optimal temporomandibular joint function, within the
limits of the functional load capacity of joint, the surgical procedure, and subject's individual circumstances.

Introduction

Post-operative physical therapy of the temporomandibular joint is a widely
accepted treatment modality following both open and arthroscopic surgical
procedures. In some textbooks, physical therapy following surgery is mentioned as being important without further explanation, while in other textbooks
a detailed description of physical therapy procedures is provided. In general,
treatment outlines used in physical therapy after orthopedic joint surgery have
been adjusted and applied to the temporomandibular joint according to its
specific anatomy, biomechanics, and arthrokinematics. Although a broad scientific basis for post-surgical physical therapy for the temporomandibular joint
is lacking, empirical and some scientific evidence has been gathered regarding
its beneficial effects.

Biologic basis for post-operative physical therapy: surgical sequelae

Even using the finest arthroscopic instruments and applying the most precise
and careful procedures and manipulations, any surgical procedure induces a
traumatic arthritis of the temporomandibular joint, independent of additional
joint pathology. A traumatic arthritis is accompanied by joint effusion, irritation
of the synovial membrane, and changes in quantity and quality of the synovial
fluid.[1] As a result, the patient will experience pain. Pain and effusion induce
reflex muscle splinting to protect the joint. Thus, the patient tends to immobilize
his (her) joint.

Immobilization has been shown to have detrimental effects on the locomotor
system. Immobilization of the primate temporomandibular joint initiates quan-

titative as well as qualitative changes in condylar cartilage.[2] After ten days of immobilization, rodent temporomandibular joints showed significant thinning of the condylar cartilage, degenerative changes, and adhesion formation.[3] Although these changes tend to be reversible, degeneration of the condylar cartilage can still be observed after eight months of remobilization.[2] Another effect of immobilization of primate temporomandibular joints is the considerable atrophy of both temporalis and masseter muscles.[4] Peri-articular connective tissue matrices lose water and glycosaminoglycans as a result of immobilization, thereby reducing the lubricational efficiency for collagen fibril-fibril friction.[5] This may lead to aberrant cross-linking, thereby reducing the range of motion.[5] Decrease of ligamental strength after immobilization has also been described.[5]

Besides these effects due to operation and immobilization, pre-existing degenerative joint pathology may have an enormous influence on masticatory function. Degenerative joint diseases and chronic arthralgia inhibit the normal use of the joint. In patients with a restricted range of mouth opening due to temporomandibular joint degenerative diseases and trauma, the temporalis and masseter muscles show significant atrophy and degeneration.[6] Masticatory muscles adapt to a restricted range of mouth opening by shortening.[7] In this way, the masticatory muscles become an additional, extra-articular, cause of mandibular movement restriction. In addition, joint effusion and pain reflexly inhibit the proper use of masticatory muscles, thus reducing maximal voluntary contraction.[8] Chronic joint pathology not only reduces masticatory muscle strength but also muscle endurance.[9] Finally, temporomandibular joint pathology inhibits joint position sense and, consequently, proper masticatory muscle coordination.[10]

Post-operative physical therapy protocols

Remarkable agreement appears to exist between proposed protocols with respect to aims and procedures of post-surgical physical therapy (tables 1, 2 and 3).[11-21] In general, the aim of post-surgical physical therapy is to reduce the side effects of the surgical procedure and to prevent secondary immobilization of the patient. This can be achieved by reducing pain and swelling, preventing re-traumatizing the joint, increasing range of motion, and improving masticatory muscle function. A second aim is to optimize masticatory function within the limits of pre-existing joint pathology, the surgical procedure, and of the individual.[11-21] In many descriptions of physical therapy programs, a pre-operative assessment is proposed.[12,14,16-18]

Pre-operative assessment

The physical therapist's pre-operative assessment is aimed at making an inventory of problems before surgery: restricted range of motion, disturbances in arthrokinematics of the temporomandibular joint that result in disturbed osteokinematics of the mandible, muscle soreness, tender and trigger points, atrophy, muscle splinting, and poor posture. In addition, the patient receives information about procedures during and following surgery. Instructions are provided concerning exercises, ice massage, and joint protection to be performed immediately after surgery.

It is important that the physical therapist is informed by the surgeon about the aim of and procedures performed during the operation, quality of the tissues encountered, range of motion under general anesthesia, and which physical therapy procedures and joint movements are (relatively) contra-indicated. It has been estimated that about 10 mm, or 30%, less than the range of motion under general anesthesia can be achieved after the physical therapy program.[13,15]

Post-operative protocol

Following a post-operative examination of the masticatory system, including assessment of range of motion, pain, swelling, muscle splinting, muscular tender and trigger points, muscle length, position sense, and muscle coordination, the post-operative physical therapy program can begin.[11-14,16,17] The program can be roughly divided into three phases:[11-17]

– immediate post-operative phase, which focuses on reducing inflammation and maintaining range of motion
– intermediate phase, about one to three weeks after the operation, in which an increase in range of motion and increased muscle control is the main objective
– late post-operative phase, about three to six weeks post-operatively, in which an increase in joint loading and masticatory function must be achieved. Another objective of this phase is that the patient is able to maintain the range of motion independent of visits to physical therapist.

In all post-operative phases, body posture is corrected, and, to achieve optimal masticatory function, home exercises are prescribed.[12-18,20]

Immediate post-operative phase (Table 1)
The objectives of the program immediate post-operatively are to reduce the effects of traumatic arthritis (i.e., reduce pain, prevent immobilization of the joint), to protect the joint from re-injury, and to promote tissue healing.

To reduce the effects from traumatic arthritis, ice application at regular intervals and transcutaneous electrical nerve stimulation are recommended in most protocols. As an addition to pain medication, pulsed ultrasound or electrostimulation are frequently proposed.[12-17,19-21] Pain inhibition may contribute to the reduction of muscle splinting. Specific exercises are given to relax

Table 1. Concise summary of post-surgical physical therapy protocols.[11-21] Immediate post-operative phase (1–7 days after surgery)

Goals	Techniques	Modalities	Home instructions*
Control inflammation			
Reduce pain	Joint distraction, grade I	Ice massage TENS ** Ultrasound, pulsed	Ice massage
Reduce swelling	Active opening and closing Joint distraction, rhythmic	Ice massage TENS Ultrasound, pulsed	Ice massage
Prevent adhesion formation	Active opening and closing	–	Move mandible frequently: vertically (hinge exercises) and horizontally (translate)
Stabilizing range of motion			
Joint mobilization	Joint distraction grade I, II	–	Move mandible frequently: vertically and horizontally
Muscle relaxation	Hold-relax	Moist heat	Hot wet towel application
Decrease joint loading	–	–	Non-chewing diet Reduce parafunctional habits

*   Exercises at home should be performed at regular intervals two to six times per day.
**   TENS = transcutaneous electrical nerve stimulation

and stretch the muscles.[11-13,15,21] Besides inhibiting the pain pulsed ultrasound also promotes tissue healing.[22] Range-of-motion exercises within the limits of pain are given to prevent adhesion formation.[11-20] Sometimes the exercises are supported by continuous passive motion devices.[23-25] Mild joint mobilization techniques, such as grade I and II joint distraction, are also given in this phase.[11-18,20] To prevent re-injury, usually the following advice is given: do not over-exercise, keep to a non-chewing diet, avoid parafunctional oral habits, prevent over-stretching of the joint by excessive yawning, talking, and laughing.[12-18,20,21] To enhance therapeutic effects, instructions are given for a home exercise program as well as the application of ice massage.[12-18,20,21]

Intermediate post-operative phase (Table 2)
In the intermediate post-operative phase pain inhibition remains important. This phase also focuses on increasing range of motion, promoting tissue healing, and increasing muscle control and mandibular awareness.[11-18,20]

For pain inhibition in this phase continuous ultrasound moist heat, current therapy, infrared radiation, or deep heat by means of shortwave diathermy are recommended.[12-17,20] Soft laser also has been proposed.[14] Modalities used in the initial phase may also be applied in this phase.

Table 2. Concise summary of post-surgical physical therapy protocols.[11-21] Intermediate post-operative phase (1–3 weeks after surgery)

Goals	Techniques	Modalities	Home instructions*
Control pain			
Reduce muscle pain	Spray and stretching Massage, frictions	Heat Ultrasound Shortwave diathermy	Gentle passive stretching Auto-massage Infrared
Reduce joint pain	Rhythmic joint distraction	Ice massage	Ice massage
Increase range of motion Improve arthrokinematics	Joint distraction grade II	–	Move mandible frequently: vertically
	Anterior glide		Move mandible frequently: horizontally
Stretch muscles	Hold-relax	–	Hold-relax techniques with tongue blades
	Transverse stretch	–	Transverse stretch
Improve muscle coordination	Rhythmic stabilization	–	Rhythmic stabilization

* Exercises at home should be performed at regular intervals two to six times per day.

Table 3. Concise summary of post-surgical physical therapy protocols.[11-21] Late post-operative phase (3–6 weeks after surgery)

Goals	Techniques	Modalities	Home instructions*
Increase range of motion	Vigorous mobilization	–	Passive stretching of mouth opening
Strengthen muscles	Isometric exercises	–	Resistance against mandibular movements
Increase functional load	–	–	Gradually start with solid food
Patient independent of therapist	Education	–	Regular exercise

* Exercises at home should be performed at regular intervals two to six times per day.

To increase the range of motion, somewhat stronger joint mobilization techniques are used. Grade II joint distraction and anterior glide techniques may be given to improve the joint's arthrokinematics. Active protrusive and latero-trusive movements are initiated. In case of muscle tightness restricting movement, muscle-stretching techniques are prescribed. Neuromuscular control is stimulated by rhythmic stabilization exercises.[11-20]

Late post-operative phase (Table 3)
In the late post-operative phase the objectives are to increase the load-bearing capacity of temporomandibular joint and masticatory muscles, and to increase the patient's independence.

Discussion

The goals of temporomandibular joint surgery and subsequent physical therapy are to achieve optimal masticatory function within the limitations of the joint, the surgical procedure, and the patient. It is obvious that a degenerative joint is limited in its functional capacity to withstand loads.[26] Surgical procedures can restore or modify this capacity only to a certain extent. The capability of the patient to cope with the restrictions of the degenerative and operated joint may play an important role in the outcome of surgery and subsequent physical therapy program.[26]

In order to achieve optimal masticatory function, pain inhibition, sufficient range of motion, and muscle control are required. Agreement exists among physical therapists as to the means by which these goals should be pursued. As a consequence, the post-operative physical therapy protocols described in different textbooks and papers are comparable.[11-21] However, this agreement is based on 'common sense' rather than on extensive scientific research results.

In general, the rationale for most physical therapy programs is that all surgical procedures, although aimed at restoring joint function and reducing pain by removal of diseased tissues, lysis of adhesions, smoothing of joint surfaces, and lavage of the joint, have a traumatizing effect to the joint. This traumatic arthritis is accompanied by swelling, joint effusion, pain, and reduction of voluntary muscle contraction.[1,8] Another important reason for post-operative physical therapy is the detrimental effect of post-surgical immobilization on joint cartilage, capsular ligament length and strength, and muscle length, power, and endurance. In addition, immobilization influences the quality of scar tissue and may enhance adhesion formation.[2-7] Probably secondary to these effects, pain may be perceived over a longer period than necessary. Therefore, pain inhibition, reduction of the features of traumatic arthritis, and mobilization of the joint are of great importance and should be undertaken early, preferably within 24 hours of the operation.

Physical therapy techniques and modalities

Without adequate inhibition of pain it is impossible to perform exercises properly, even for the best-motivated patient. Therefore, adequate pain medication must be given post-operatively. Additional ice application by means of ice massage, coldpacks, or ice chips reduces pain considerably.[27] Reduction of pain will improve the range of motion and the patient's confidence. Moreover, ice application reduces intra-articular temperature significantly, thereby reducing inflammation.[28] Ice should not be used in cases of cold hypersensitivity or poor circulation, and care should be taken not to apply too much ice.[29]

To promote tissue healing, and to reduce inflammation, swelling, and pain in the immediate post-operative phase, pulsed ultrasound is frequently proposed.[12-17,19,20] The mechanism underlying its effects is thought to be the rhythmic pressure changes within the different tissues caused by the ultrasound waves.[30,31] Enhanced quality and quantity of tissue healing due to ultrasound was established in an animal study.[22] Other perceived effects of ultrasound are not beyond discussion, since these effects appear largely to be placebo effects.[31-33]

Also in the immediate post-operative phase, transcutaneous electrical nerve stimulation is applied to reduce pain. The effects of pain inhibition are currently explained by gate-control mechanisms and release of endorphins in the central nervous system.[34] However, scientific evidence for the effectiveness of transcutaneous electrical nerve stimulation in reducing pain is limited, and, again, placebo effects may be of considerable importance.[31,35]

In most post-operative protocols, in the intermediate and the late phases after surgery some kind of thermal agent for elevating tissue temperature is proposed. These agents include moist heat (warm towels, hotpacks), continuous ultrasound, or shortwave diathermy. The rationale for these applications is that heat reduces pain and muscle tension.[36] Furthermore, raising collagen temperature may increase its extensibility, which may have beneficial effects during stretching procedures.[37] However, these modalities have been shown to increase temperature even intra-articularly.[27,28] In degenerative joints, elevation of temperature may enhance activities of articular-cartilage-degrading enzymes;[38] moreover elevating synovial fluid temperature may make the joint vulnerable to lubrication failure.[39] Therefore, heat can be beneficial in reducing pain and muscle tension but should not be applied over the joint. Other pain-modulating modalities proposed include infrared radiation, contrast application of heat and ice, soft laser, and galvanic stimulation. These modalities and new modalities should be tested for their clinical effectiveness in treating post-surgery patients before incorporating them in post-surgical physical therapy protocols.

The aim of increasing the mandibular range of motion is to achieve a functional mouth opening (when possible) of 35-40 mm interincisal distance.[11,13,15,16,18] Interestingly, this is about the range of motion most patients achieve in the several studies undergoing post-operative rehabilitation.[19,20,23,25]

However, it is possible that measures to increase the range of mouth opening may also result in an increase in pain in the immediate post-operative phase. Therefore, in this phase a restricted mouth opening must be temporarily accepted. Range of motion exercises should be performed gently, i.e., without enhancing traumatic arthritis or overstretching operated tissues.

Austin and Shupe showed that the increase in maximal mouth opening of patients who underwent temporomandibular joint surgery followed by physical therapy was significantly larger than that of patients without post-surgical physical therapy.[20] Physical therapy consisted of application of ice, ultrasound, electrotherapy, moist heat, joint distraction techniques, range of motion exercises, hinge exercises, and lifestyle education. After about two weeks joint distraction and isometric exercises were added, and after about 3 to 4 weeks translation techniques were given in addition to wooden tongue blade exercises. In a study conducted by Braun, only subjects undergoing temporomandibular joint surgery with a grossly delayed recovery of mouth opening and considerable arthralgia one month after surgery were given post-surgical physical therapy.[19] The control group consisted of subjects with a normal or a rapid recovery after surgery, mildly restricted mouth opening, and minimal or moderate arthralgia on function. The maximal mouth opening in the physical therapy group showed a significantly larger increase in range of motion (11.8 mm) compared with the increase in range of motion in the control group (8.8 mm). The mean range of motion did not significantly differ between the two groups. Reported pain reduced considerably in the therapy group. It was suggested that restricted joint mobility may be one of the factors enhancing arthralgia and dysfunction. The physical therapy program consisted of superficial heat, ultrasound, jaw range of motion exercises, and joint mobilization techniques. The use of pain medication was not assessed in this study.

Joint distraction techniques are most frequently advocated in order to increase range of motion. It has been shown that specific joint mobilization techniques increase range of motion and reduce pain significantly, even in subjects with severe destruction of the temporomandibular joint from rheumatoid arthritis and ankylosing spondylitis.[40] In another study, muscle stretching and strengthening within pain-free limits of the joint also increased range of motion significantly in subjects whose temporomandibular joints were severely affected by rheumatoid arthritis and ankylosing spondylitis.[9] The most effective treatment protocol for increasing range of motion, e.g. joint distraction techniques, active range of motion exercises, muscle strengthening exercises, or a combination of these techniques, remains to be established, however.

In orthopedics, continuous passive motion has been successfully applied post-operatively to reduce the detrimental effects of immobilization and to increase range of motion. Recently, continuous passive motion has been introduced in the post-operative care of the temporomandibular joint patient.[23-25] Some continuous passive motion devices have been shown to be effective in increasing range of motion.[23,24] In a small clinical trial, maximal interincisal opening in two groups of temporomandibular joint surgery patients was evaluated.[23] The experimental group received a continuous passive motion device which opened and closed the mouth at a speed of one cycle each 45 seconds. The control group did not receive continuous passive motion. Neither group received additional physical therapy. The post-operative increase of maximal opening was significantly larger in the experimental group (19 mm) compared with the control group (4 mm). Moreover, post-surgically the mean maximal interincisal distance was significantly greater in the experimental group (47 mm) that in the control group (25 mm), while before operation the maximal interincisal distance did not differ significantly between the groups.[23] In a recent study, temporomandibular joint surgery patients were treated with a standard physical therapy program and additionally a group of patients received continuous passive motion, which initiated mainly translatory movements.[24] In both groups maximal mouth opening increased significantly, but for the continuous passive motion group the mean mouth opening (43 mm) was significantly greater than that of the control group (40.5 mm), while pre-operatively the maximal mouth opening did not differ significantly between the groups. Favorable effects of continuous passive motion have even been reported in patients with multiple temporomandibular joint surgeries.[25] Thus, continuous passive motion seems to be effective post-operatively in increasing the range of motion, although it is not clear whether it is more effective than post-surgical physical therapy. In addition, it remains to be established what kind of continuous passive motion should be given (rotation, translation, or both), and with what frequency and speed.

Temporomandibular joint pathology considerably affects the masticatory muscles.[6] Masticatory muscles adapt (shorten) to a restricted range of motion dictated by joint or peri-articular tissues, and in severely restricted joints muscle fiber degeneration may occur.[7] These effects may be more pronounced when joint pathology exists for a longer period of time before the operation. If the goal of temporomandibular joint surgery is to increase the range of motion by lysis of intra-articular adhesions, it is most important to stretch the masticatory muscles post-operatively in order to gain the full range of motion possible intra-articularly. Muscle-stretching techniques include static stretching, hold-relax techniques, and contract-relax antagonist-contract techniques.[41] Of these techniques, the latter has been shown to be the most effective in gaining range of motion.[41]

Furthermore, as a result of joint pathology, the masticatory muscles tend to protect the joint. When this situation exists for a long period of time, these muscles may become overloaded and be a source of pain themselves.[42] Pre- and post-operatively, tender and trigger points are often found in the masticatory muscles. Stretching these muscles combined with spraying techniques may reduce these tender and trigger points.[42]

Degenerative diseases of the temporomandibular joint as well as of other synovial joints impair joint position sense.[10,43] For proper functioning, mandibular position sense is needed to move the jaw in the appropriate direction. Post-operative physical therapy can be hindered by a grossly impaired joint position sense. When the patient is not able to control mandibular movements due to reduced joint position sense, it is recommended to regain this sense by rhythmic stabilization exercises and by providing visual feedback by using a mirror.[11-16]

Little attention is given to the rehabilitation of muscle strength in the different protocols. Only one protocol, describing physical therapy after or-thognatic surgery, provides detailed information concerning muscle strength training.[44] The length of the post-operative immobilization period (one to eight weeks) has consequences for masticatory muscle strength. Most temporo-mandibular joint surgery procedures do not have such a long immobilization period, however.

Controversy exists regarding which movements to perform and which to avoid. For example, Austin and Shupe favor hinge exercises because translatory movements are considered harmful for the joint,[20] while McCarty and Darnell strongly propose translation of the temporomandibular joint post-operatively.[24] When evaluating the arthrokinematics of the healthy temporomandibular joint, a relatively fixed ratio between rotation and translation exists, and these movements seem to be mutually dependent.[45-48] With this in mind, the discus-sion whether rotation should be preferred over translation or visa versa seems futile. However, the arthrokinematics of the pathologic joint may differ con-siderably from that of a healthy joint, which makes the discussion interesting again. Future research needs to evaluate the benefits of translation and rotation or a combination of both.

General agreement exists concerning a soft diet after surgery. Non-chewing diets are prescribed in order to prevent joint overloading. A gradual return to a normal diet should be strictly monitored, since it cannot be expected that an immediate return to a normal diet after a six-week-long non-chewing diet will be without problems. Other activities that overload the joint, such as excessive yawning, nail biting, gum chewing, and other parafunctional habits should be prevented. One study suggests that too much laughing is harmful to the temporomandibular joint and, consequently, should be avoided.[20] However, this advice should be modified to "do not open your mouth widely when laughing but laugh as much as possible". Most temporomandibular joint patients probably do well with a little bit of laughter.

Design of a post-surgical physical therapy program

A physical therapy program can be designed based on the patient's signs and symptoms, or on the length of the post-surgical period. Both strategies have advantages and disadvantages.

A sign-dependent design adjusts the intensity and progress of the physical therapy to the demands and needs of the patient. Evaluation of the therapeutic measures and their combined effects on the different tissues is made constantly, and the therapeutic measures are adjusted accordingly. An advantage of this strategy is that overloading is recognized immediately, and appropriate measures can be taken (i.e., decrease in exercise intensity, and reduction in joint loading). A major disadvantage is the risk that frequent reports of pain or discomfort may enhance somatic fixation and progression towards a chronic pain syndrome.

A time-dependent design (cookbook recipe) has the advantage that the different therapeutic activities are applied within a certain time span, which results in a highly standardized and clear protocol. A disadvantage is that one can hardly adapt the program to responses from the patient or the joint. Pre-existing joint pathology may influence greatly the load the joint can bear and the functional performance of the joint. Probably a combination of both strategies is needed to gain optimal effects.

A problem in reviewing the protocols is that for each the time span of the immediate, intermediate, and final post-operative phases differs. Differences in clinical experience of surgeon and physical therapist, sign interpretation, and healing time of the various tissues involved in surgery may explain the variation in time span between the protocols. Much research needs to be done in this area.

Three sessions of half an hour of post-surgical physical therapy per week is not enough to achieve sufficient progress. A post-surgical physical therapy program is not complete unless patients receive instructions concerning home exercises. Patients should be instructed in ice massage and superficial heat application in order to control pain and swelling, and in addition patients should be assigned exercises to increase range of motion, and coordinate, stretch, and strengthen muscles to enable them to continue their therapy independently.

Conclusions

Post-surgical physical therapy can effectively increase mandibular range of motion. In general, the physical therapy program should start as soon as possible after surgery. The design of the program should be aimed at the different tissues involved in surgery and those surrounding the joint. It should reduce post-operative traumatic arthritis and prevent immobilization. Eventually, post-operative physical therapy aims at optimal temporomandibular joint function within the limits of the joint and surgical procedure.

The modalities for post-surgical physical therapy need to be evaluated to optimize the effectiveness of the program. Currently used post-operative physical therapy programs are based on available knowledge and are derived from the different fields of medicine. However, programs may need to be adapted according to future research results.

References

1   Pinals RS. Traumatic arthritis and allied conditions. In McCarty DJ, Koopman WJ (eds), Arthritis and allied conditions 12th Ed. Philadelphia: Lea & Febiger, 1993; 1521

2   Glineburg RW, Laskin DM, Blaustein DI. The effects of immobilization on the primate temporomandibular joint: A histological and histochemical study. J Oral Maxillofac Surg 1982; 40:3

3   Lydiatt DD, Davis LF. The effects of immobilization on the rabbit temporomandibular joint. J Oral Maxillofac Surg 1985; 43:188

4   Mayo KH, Ellis E, Carlson DS. Histochemical analysis of the masseter and temporalis muscles in Macaca Mulatta after mandibular advancement using rigid and nonrigid fixation. J Oral Maxillofac Surg 1990; 48:381

5   Ellis E, Carlson DS. The effects of mandibular immobilization on the masticatory system. A review. Clin Plast Surg 1989; 19:133

6   El-Labban NG, Harris M, Hopper C, Barber P. Degenerative changes in masseter and temporalis muscles in limited mouth opening and TMJ ankylosis. J Oral Pathol Med 1990; 19:423

7   El-Labban NG, Cannif JP. Ultrastructural findings of muscle degeneration in oral submucous fibrosis. J Oral Pathol 1985; 14:709

8   Young A, Stokes M, Iles JF. Effects of joint pathology on muscle. Clin Orthop Rel Res 1987; 219:21

9   Tegelberg Å, Kopp S. Short-term effect of physical training on temporomandibular joint disorders in individuals with rheumatoid arthritis and ankylosing spondylitis. Acta Odontol Scand 1988; 46:49

10 Isacsson G, Isberg A, Persson A. Loss of directional orientation of lower jaw movements in persons with internal derangement of the temporomandibular joint. Oral Surg Oral Med Oral Pathol 1988; 66:8

11 Plante D. Postoperative physical therapy. In: Keith I, Alexander D (eds). Surgery of the temporomandibular joint. Boston: Blackwell, 1988; 263

12 Uriell P. Bertolucci L, Swaffer C. Physical therapy in the postoperative management of temporomandibular joint arthroscopic surgery. J Craniomandibular Pract 1989; 7:27

13 Bertolucci L, Uriell P, Swaffer C. Postoperative physical therapy in temporomandibular joint arthroplasty. J Craniomandibular Pract 1989; 7:214

14 Bertolucci L. Physical therapy post-arthroscopic TMJ management (Update). J Craniomandibular Pract 1992; 10:130

15 Rocabado M. Physical therapy for the postsurgical TMJ patient. J Craniomandib Disord Facial Oral Pain 1989; 3:75

16 Dunn J. Physical Therapy. In: Kaplan AS, Assael LA (eds). Temporomandibular disorders: diagnosis and treatment. Philadelphia: Saunders, 1991; 455

17 Eggleton TM, Langton DP. Post-arthroscopic physical rehabilitation of the temporomandibular joint. In: Thomas M, Bronstein SL (eds). Arthroscopy of the temporomandibular joint. Philadelphia: Saunders, 1991; 294

18 Wilk BR, McCain JP. Rehabilitation of the temporomandibular joint after arthroscopic surgery. Oral Surg Oral Med Oral Pathol 1992; 73:531

19 Braun BL. The effect of physical therapy intervention on incisal opening after temporomandibular joint surgery. Oral Surg Oral Med Oral Pathol 1987; 64:544

20 Austin BD, Shupe SM. The role of physical therapy in recovery after temporomandibular joint surgery. J Oral Maxillofac Surg 1993; 51:495

21 Dijkstra PU, de Bont LGM, Boering G. Physiotherapy protocol following arthroscopy of the temporomandibular joint. 10th Congress of the Eur Assoc Cranio Max Fac Surg, Brussels, 1990; abstr. 261

22 Byl NN, McKenzie AL, West JM, et al. Low-dose ultrasound on wound healing: a controled study with Yucatan pigs. Arch Phys Med Rehabil 1992; 73:656

23 Sebastian MH, Moffet MC. The effects of continuous passive motion on the temporomandibular joint after surgery. Oral Surg Oral Med Oral Pathol 1989; 67:644

24 McCarty WL, Darnell MW. Rehabilitation of the temporomandibular joint through the application of motion. J Craniomandibular Pract 1993; 11:298

25 Fontenot MG. Continuous passive motion following total temporomandibular joint arthroplasty J Oral Maxillofac Surg 1989; 47 (Suppl), 138

26 Stegenga B. Temporomandibular joint osteoarthrosis. Diagnostic and treatment outcome assessment. Thesis, University of Groningen, The Netherlands, 1991

27 Bugaj R. The cooling, analgesic, and rewarming effects of ice massage on localized skin. Phys Ther 1975; 55:11

28 Oosterveld FGJ, Rassker JJ, Jacobs JWG, Overmars HJA. The effect of local heat and cold therapy on the intraarticular and skin temperature of the knee. Arthritis Rheum 1992; 35:146

29 Michlovitz SL. Cryotherapy: The use of cold as a therapeutic agent. In: Michlovitz SL, Wolf SL (eds). Thermal agents in rehabilitation. Philadelphia: Davis Co, 1986; 73

30 Ziskin MC, Michlovitz SL. Therapeutic ultrasound. In: Michlovitz SL, Wolf SL (eds). Thermal agents in rehabilitation. Philadelphia: Davis Co, 1986; 141

31 Mohl ND, Ohrbach RK, Crow HC, Gross AJ. Devices for the diagnosis and treatment of temporomandibular disorders. Part III: Thermography, ultrasound, electrical stimulation, and electromyographic biofeedback. J Prosthet Dent 1990; 63:472

32 Hashish I, Hai HK, Harvey W, et al. Reduction of postoperative pain and swelling by ultrasound treatment: a placebo effect. Pain 1988; 33:303

33 Hashish I, Harvey W, Harris M. Anti-inflammatory effects of ultrasound therapy: evidence for a major placebo effect. Br J Rheumatol 1986; 25:77

34 Mannheimer JS, Lampe GN. Clinical transcutaneous electrical nerve stimulation. Philadelphia: Davis Co, 1986

35 Moystad A, Krogstad BS, Larheim TA. Transcutaneous nerve stimulation in a group of patients with rheumatic disease involving the temporomandibular joint. J Prosthet Dent 1990; 64:596

36 Michlovitz SL. Biophysical principles of heating and superficial heat agents. In: Michlovitz SL, Wolf SL (eds). Thermal agents in rehabilitation. Philadelphia: Davis Co, 1986; 99

37 Mannheimer JS. Physical therapy: concepts in evaluation and treatment of the upper quarter. Therapeutic modalities. In: Kraus SL (ed). TMJ disorders: management of the craniomandibular complex. New York: Churchill Livingstone, 1988; 311

38 Harris ED, McCroskery PA. The influence of temperature and fibril stability on degradation of cartilage collagen by rheumatoid synovial collagenase. New Engl J Med 1974; 290:1

39 Webb A, Stachowiak PL, O'Neill PL, Batchelor AW. The effects of temperature changes and arthritis on the lubricating properties of synovial fluid. J Orthop Rheumatol 1993; 6:81

40 Sandführ K, Linke M, Witteck J. Manuelle Therapie entzündlich befallene Kiefergelenke. Mannuelle Medizin 1988; 26:35

41 Etnyer BR, Abraham LD. Gains in range of ankle dorsiflexion using three popular stretching techniques. Am J Phys Med 1986; 65:189

42 Travel JG, Simons DG. Myofascial pain and dysfunction. The trigger point manual. Baltimore: Williams & Wilkins, 1983

43 Barret DS, Cobb AG, Bentley G. Joint proprioception in normal, osteoarthrotic and replaced knees. J Bone Joint Surg [Br] 1991; 73-B:53

44 Bell WH, Gonyea W, Finn RA, et al. Muscular rehabilitation after orthognathic surgery. Oral Surg Oral Med Oral Pathol 1983; 56:229

45 Merlini L, Palla S. The relationship between condylar rotation and anterior translation in healthy and clicking temporomandibular joints. Schweiz Monatss Zahnmed 1988; 98:1191

46 Falkenström Ch. Biomechanical design of a total temporomandibular joint replacement. Thesis, Technical University of Enschede, the Netherlands, 1993

47 Osborne JW. The temporomandibular ligament and the articular eminence as constraints during jaw opening. J Oral Rehabil 1989; 16:323

48 Dijkstra PU. Temporomandibular joint osteoarthrosis and joint mobility. Thesis, University of Groningen, The Netherlands, 1993

Management of Temporomandibular
Joint Degenerative Diseases
ed. by B. Stegenga & L.G.M. de Bont
© 1996 Birkhäuser Verlag Basel/Switzerland

Correction of temporomandibular joint ankylosis resulting from earlier surgery

Robert B. MacIntosh

Department of Dentistry and Oral and Maxillofacial Surgery, Sinai Hospital of Detroit, Detroit, Michigan, USA

Summary: Experience with patients with temporomandibular joint ankylosis resulting from earlier surgery suggests that the difference between severe fibrous restriction and true ankylosis is academic, that ankylosis is more frequently encountered after removal of alloplasts than while they are still in place, that costochondral grafting without concomitant placement of a dermal interface leads to a rather high rate of re-ankylosis, and that programmed physical therapy is not a major factor in determining the ultimate success in this group of patients.

Introduction

Experiences, good and bad, have led the author to adopt a four-point teaching philosophy consistent with the current knowledge:

– the clinician should make every attempt possible to manage the sympto-matic temporomandibular joint patient non-surgically
– if the joint must be opened, the surgeon should make every attempt possible to salvage the normal disc and normal condyle
– if the disc and/or the condyle cannot be salvaged because of displacement, scarification, fracture, atrophy, or whatever other intractable damage, the native elements should be removed and replaced with autogenous substitutes
– with infrequent exception, all polymerized condyle, disc, and fossa substitutes, and most metallic alloy substitutes, should be removed and replaced with autogenous substitutes.

These considerations are pertinent to the prevention and management of temporomandibular joint ankylosis.

Historically, ankylosis of the temporomandibular joint has several etiolo-gies, but, in the American experience of the past two decades, ankylosis resulting from repeated surgical invasion of the joint for correction of disc and/or condylar abnormalities has become increasingly prominent. Most of these difficulties reflect the scarification resulting from the intense inflamma-tory reaction incited by alloplastic discs. Severe restriction of movement is recognized also as a reaction around total joint prostheses. Not all ankylosis in the modern context, however, results from the placement of alloplasts. Various non-alloplastic arthroplasty procedures, particularly when repeated, can also engender severe fibrosis, degeneration and impaired regeneration of normal anatomy, and resultant restriction of movement.

This chapter reflects the philosophy that reconstruction with autogenous tissues offers the best possibility for lysis of temporomandibular joint restriction on grounds of both physiology and clinical experience. The literature reflects successful elimination of ankylosis of more classic etiology through the use of alloplasts; for the great majority of today's patients in their younger years, however, for whom restitution of normal joint function and maintenance of good mandibular position and occlusion are paramount, there is no convincing evidence to refute the superiority of autogenous tissues in their repairs.

Etiology of fibrous and true ankylosis

In many cases, the distinction between true ankylosis (i.e., absolute continuity of bone across an articulation) and severe fibrous restriction of articular movement is academic. The discomfort, the compromise in mastication, and the destruction of the dentition, can be devastating regardless of the histology. Surgical elimination of the problem demands the same precision and care, and entails essentially the same surgical frustrations, since the operative morbidities and chance for re-ankylosis pertain whether the pathologic tissue is fibrous or osseous.

Discoplasty

The chief indication for this procedure is "closed-lock", which denotes impedance to condylar anterior excursion by fixed, or at least frequent, anterior displacement of the disc, and discomfort on condylar excursion. The encouraging results in alleviation of symptoms reported during the resurgence of this technique some two decades ago have not been consistently substantiated in patients examined over protracted periods of time. The repositioned disc is often too thin to withstand normal functional pressure, so that discoplasty occasionally fails completely, regressing past resurgent discomfort and "locking" to severe fibrous restriction and/or bony union.

Discectomy

The indications proposed for discectomy are essentially those for discoplasty, i.e., intractable closed-lock, and pain associated with this limitation. Henny, one of discectomy's strongest proponents in the 1940s and 1950s, subsequently abandoned the procedure. Most of the reports regarding discectomy in the American literature, however, do not condemn it, but, in fact, support it.[1-4]

Recently, probably out of frustration with other disc salvaging or replacement techniques, discectomy seems to have regained support among American surgeons. The author's own experience, however, gained from observation of patients over the medium- and long-terms, has been all but uniformly negative. Once the disc, which is designed to absorb the deforming forces of muscle contraction, is removed, one can expect the approximating bony surfaces of the articular eminence and the condyle either to eburnate, hopefully, with the development of new cortical bone, or, discouragingly, to become further abraded, inflamed, and, potentially, to fibrose, scarify, and occasionally ossify.

High condylectomy

In high condylectomy, or "condylar shave", a broad surface of medullary bone lies exposed across the articulating surface of the condyle once 2-4 mm of overlying irregular or eroded cortical surface is removed.[2] In most cases, particularly those in which a generally normal disc remains, the condylar head can be expected to regain a cortical surface, albeit in many cases with unusual contour, covered with articular cartilage. In a few instances, however, the decorticated surface does not heal as desired, but, instead, becomes more inflamed and fibrotically adherent to the disc and/or other elements of the articulation. This tissue, too, occasionally ossifies to develop a true ankylosis.

Failed alloplastic devices

The patient with the failed alloplast undoubtedly constitutes the greatest problem in temporomandibular joint surgery today. The essential destruction phenomenon is the now well-recognized foreign body giant cell reaction and osteoclastic activity associated with mechanical disintegration of the device.[5] In clinical terms, deterioration of the device results in destruction of any of the condylar elements and, if the inflammatory response is severe enough, significant fibrous and/or bony restriction of the articulation.

The total joint prostheses can also provoke severe soft tissue restriction, and even bony obliteration of the articulation. These devices have found most common application as replacements for the articular elements following ablative surgery or as end-stage substitutes following a cascade of failed earlier attempts at alloplastic reconstruction. The most significant cause of failure of these devices is directly analogous to that which occurs around the alloplastic disc. Loosening of the metal condyle seems to be infrequent, but progressive fibrosis around the condyle, and between it and the alloplastic fossa, accounts occasionally for a gradual decrease in the range of mandibular motion.

True or pseudoankylosis can ensue even after removal of the alloplasts. This is not an infrequent occurrence in the author's experience, and is at least partially related to the demonstrated ability of residual alloplast in the wound to provoke an exaggerated healing response.[6]

To date, there has not been an alloplast devised for joint replacement that does not carry the potential for inciting an undesired inflammatory response.[7] Disintegration seems to be limited not simply to the polymer alloplasts. The orthopedic literature describes microfragmentation and soft tissue reaction around whole metal articulations as well.

Failed autogenous grafts

Though not as frequently encountered, ankylosis following invasive auto- genous reconstruction of the temporomandibular articulation is recognized.[8] Scarification is acceptable, indeed even desirable, in the context of developing a viable, durable, interface between condyle and fossa, but there is no guarantee that such a healing response will not fuse the reconstructive elements. The ankylosis or re-ankylosis ensuing subsequent to the replacement of autogenous disc or condylar substitutes can be just as severe as that from any other cause.

Management considerations

Eradication of ankylosis mandates recognition of particulars not quite as significant in other temporomandibular joint procedures. Firstly, the potential anatomical hazards can be severe, particularly in children. If the ankylotic mass extends far medially, great care is necessary to avoid the internal maxillary, the middle meningeal, and even the internal carotid arteries. Fusion to the roof of the fossa, particularly in the absence of any residual disc, or to the deeper region of the petrous portion of the temporal bone, puts both the middle cranial fossa and the acoustic branch of the VIIIth nerve at hazard if sectioning through the redundant bone is at all injudicious. Access to even lateral mass alone can be problematic in severe cases, and temporal flap exposure is often advisable, even mandatory.

The second particular consideration is the tendency toward re-ankylosis post-operatively. This potential is strongest in children. Effective lysis of tem- poromandibular joint ankylosis entails, in the author's opinion, removal of at least 2 cm of bone across the ossified site. Often, the transection is best executed at a position inferior to the original articulation to obviate inadvertent perforation of the middle cranial fossa and encroachment on other important structures.

Reconstruction options

If the ankylosis is not overly severe, and/or is not completely osseous, and/or is limited to intra-articular boundaries, separation and removal of bone at the site of original articulation is often possible. This resculpturing is enhanced by the presence of any residual disc within the mass of redundant bone. In such cases, placement of an interpositonal soft tissue graft is advisable to inhibit re-ossification. There is little role for alloplasts in this circumstance, in the author's opinion. The only realistic choice is between autogenous or bank tissues.

In severe cases in which masses of extraneous bone pertain, and particularly in instances in which re-ankylosis has occurred following earlier attempts at elimination of bony union, any residual semblance of normal anatomy is totally absent. In these situations, resection of medio-laterally wide blocks of bone, more than 2 cm in height and often inferior to the original articulation, will most frequently require ultimate restitution of hard tissue. Replacement of the lost bone is best accomplished on a delayed basis, in the author's opinion. When this need is evident, the option of artificial replacement of condyle and/or ramus still exists. If such a device is to be used, the necessity for autogenous disc replacement is obviated because such tissues will not withstand the force of the metallic condyle. The concomitant placement of a metallic fossa is advisable, since the ability of the bone alone to withstand the functional stresses of a metal condyle beyond the short-term is questionable. In addition to the problem of limited adaptability of such devices at the surgical site, their absolute lack of remodeling capacity, and problems with patient comfort, there are also reports of re-ankylosis around such devices. Many experienced surgeons will testify to the extreme difficulty of freeing such devices from a re-ankylotic mass of bone when it occurs. For these reasons, reconstruction with autogenous or bank bone seems eminently preferable to any artificial device.

Autogenous substitutes

The autogenous soft tissues described for interposition following lysis of ankylosis include temporalis muscle, masseter muscle, temporalis fascia, pericranium, fascia lata, epidermis, and dermis. Costal cartilage, auricular cartilage, and the fibrocartilaginous tissues over the ilium have been utilized as hard tissue substitutes.

Despite ease of access and its proximity to the articulation, temporalis muscle, either as a free graft or pedicled, would seem to have limitations as a substitute.[9] When it functions as it is meant to function, muscle is among the strongest tissues in the body. When it is not under active contraction, it is among the flimsiest. All rotated muscle is known to atrophy even when included in large flaps with intact large-bore vessels. It can certainly be expected to undergo no less atrophy as a free graft. Additionally, there have been reports of rather severe discomfort following transportation of muscle into the articulation, suggesting the survival of sensory nerve tissue within the muscle which reacts undesirably to functional stresses put upon it.

Temporalis fascia, pericranium, or fascia lata in single layers cannot function as discs, and it seems improbable that such tissues would prove barriers to any re-ankylotic tendency. When folded in layers sufficiently thick to form a seemingly adequate impediment to re-ossification, one can only speculate as to the likelihood of neovascular penetration of this very dense tissue.

Cartilage would seem to be an ideal tissue for impedance of re-ankylosis, but successful attempts to model costal cartilage to the contours of the fossa, and to stabilize it appropriately have not been described convincingly in the literature. Härle has described the efficacy of bank cartilage in reconstruction of the joint, and this experience attests to the at least biologic legitimacy of its use in ankylosis.[10] Ideally, auricular cartilage should prove applicable because of ease of harvest and adaptability to intra-articular contours. Even under optimal circumstances, fixation of such grafts can be difficult, and the cartilage often proves too thin to withstand masticatory forces. Yih et al. have recently described other difficulties with this tissue in vivo.[11]

The dermal graft appears to be the preferred autogenous device for substitution of the disc by most surgeons today. It is the one autogenous tissue used for disc replacement that finds strong substantiation in the laboratory animal.[12] Dermis used in double thickness fashion has proved preferable in terms of strength, adaptability to the fossa, and survivability. The most significant potential disadvantage of the dermal graft is that of epidermal cyst development, which has occurred in two reported cases.[8]

The use of full-thickness epidermis, despite its having been reported in the literature, would seem to be prohibited by the potential for cyst development. The use of lyophilized tissues, most notably dura, as disc replacement has fallen into favor primarily because of the lack of demonstrated long-term efficacy.

Unquestionably, the hard tissue which has found most frequent, long-standing, and successful application as replacement of the mandibular condyle and portions of the ramus has been the costochondral graft.[12,13] The recognized advantages of the costochondral graft are its ready adaptability to the confines of even the distorted articular fossa, its low tendency toward ankylosis, and its response, it terms of strength, form, and overall dimension, to the forces put upon it. Consistency in these regards with the use of any other hard tissue element has not been convincingly reported in the literature. Re-ankylosis of the costochondral graft is an infrequent event, but when it does occur it can be just as severe as ankylosis from any other source.

The employment of the sternoclavicular graft, first espoused 90 years ago by Lexer and more recently by other authors,[14] holds certain theoretical advantages over other hard tissues and may prove to be an effective substitute for the destroyed temporomandibular articulation. Whether this procedure, with its complexity and potential donor site morbidities, will prove superior to the long-established efficacy of the costochondral graft, particularly in cases of ankylosis, awaits long-term evaluation.

Disadvantages common to all autogenous tissues are the morbidities of their donor sites, and the difficulty in demonstrating their host site statuses with imaging because of the lucency of cartilage and the soft tissues, and the irregularity of the bone-cartilage interface. The singular advantages of autogenous tissues, which make them consistently preferable to the use of alloplastic devices in the management of ankylosis, are their immediate biocompatibility, their adaptability to the bizarre anatomy and unexpected anatomical circumstances related to ankylosis, and the lack of mystery in their long-term fate. Even in the event of re-ankylosis, bone will react as bone and soft tissue as soft tissue, so that the physiologic difficulties can be anticipated and appropriately addressed.

Surgical protocols

The approach to lysis of ankylosis in this author's hands varies depending on the circumstances evoking the bony union. Patients with ankylosis developed subsequent to discoplasty, discectomy, or condylectomy, or those having experienced re-ankylosis following lysis of ankylosis of any etiology, undergo ablation of the ankylosis and concomitant interpositioning of autogenous soft tissues. Those patients suffering severe restriction of joint mobility as a result of alloplastic disc or total joint implantation undergo lysis, removal of the alloplasts, and extirpation of all reactive tissue. Placement of autogenous tissues is deferred, however, for at least 12 months.

Immediate reconstruction

If static or worsening jaw immobility persists for a period of at least 12 months subsequent to non-alloplastic arthroplasty or lysis of ankylosis, as determined both clinically and by imaging, surgical correction should be undertaken. The year-long period of observation is admittedly arbitrary, but one can reasonably expect, in an otherwise healthy individual, that post-surgical neovascularization, maximum elasticization of fibrosis, and restitution of regional muscle tone will have transpired after that period, affording optimum conditions for additional surgery. Operating before that time exposes the patient to additional traumatic insult that may aggravate physiologic healing and prove additionally detrimental. An autogenous interface, preferably dermis, is placed concomitantly and generally proves sufficient in discouraging re-ankylosis. Care must be taken to cover the entire area of exposed bone, both superiorly and inferiorly, with the interposed tissue.

As mentioned earlier, this protocol, to date, has rarely failed to inhibit re-ankylosis in the author's hands. In some patients, eradication of the ankylotic block of the minimum 2 cm vertical dimension previously mentioned, particularly in unilateral cases, may not significantly disturb either mandibular position or occlusion. In those individuals in whom it is evident that hard tissue reconstruction will be necessary, however, such care is deferred for at least 12 months. Experience has shown that placement of bone at the first lysis operation encourages re-ankylosis.

Delayed reconstruction

In those patients experiencing ankylosis subsequent to undergoing alloplastic replacement of any of the articular elements, the effective therapeutic approach is more protracted. Because persistence of the destructive tissue associated with alloplasts can be expected to destroy any autogenous tissues placed into a field of their incomplete removal, and because the surgeon can never be absolutely certain that he has removed all pathologic material, the appropriate protocol in these patients calls for aggressive ablation of the ankylotic tissue and all foreign and reactive material in one session, and subsequent reconstruction with autogenous tissues only at a date at least 12 months later.

It is prudent for the surgeon, at the time of definitive reconstruction, to first investigate the articular site, visually, tactilly, and with frozen-section evaluation, prior to harvesting the grafts. If, as a result of these inspections, there is evidence of residual reactive tissue, all such material should be removed, the wound closed, and definitive care once again deferred. If these examinations give no evidence of ongoing pathology, the grafts are harvested, and reconstruction undertaken.

In many patients in the delayed group, and some in the immediate group discussed above, interposition of an autogenous soft tissue graft is not sufficient to restore acceptable joint anatomy. The severity of condylar destruction or the magnitude of the deformity resulting from lysis of the ankylosis is often sufficiently severe to mandate hard tissue restitution of the condyle and/or ramus. At the second intervention in this delayed group, therefore, an autogenous costochondral graft is brought to position at the time the soft tissue transplant is placed.

This two-stage protocol for reconstruction demands patience and tolerance of all concerned, but experience has shown it to be effective in avoiding extensive reconstruction efforts that subsequently might be compromised. The interlude between surgeries obliges the patient to function with a significant malocclusion and some degree of discomfort in many cases. Supportive care, including occlusal splinting to facilitate mastication, may be necessary during this period.

Experience with the operative protocols

Material and methods

Tables 1 and 2 outline the series of patients treated under the described protocols. Certain of the early patients operated under the delayed protocol were operated earlier than the later-mandated 12-month interval. The term "severe fibrous restriction" was used to describe mouth opening limited to 10 mm or less, in patients in whom imaging did not demonstrate continuous ossification across either of the articulations. How many patients operated

Table 1. True ankylosis

Patient	Sex	Number of previous surgeries	Type of previous surgeries	Uni/bi lateral	Reconstructive protocol	Tissue	Outcome
BM	F	4	1,3,2,4	B	D	DG	S
AA	F	2	1,2,4	B	D	DG	S
TH	F	19	1,3,4,6,5,6	B	D	DG/CCG	Q
TK	F	4	1,4,6	B	D	DG/CCG	S
GW	F	21	1,3,2,4	U	D	DG/CCG	S
LC	F	3	2,4,6	B	D	DG/CCG	S
RS	M	1	1	B	I	DG/CCG	S
PK	F	1	1	U	I	DG	U
JK	F	1	2	B	I	DG	S
TK	F	2	1,2	B	I	DG	S
JK	F	2	1,3	B	I	DG	Q
CC	F	4	1,2,3	B	I	DG	S
KN	F	1	7,8	U	I	DG	S
RF	F	1	7,8	U	I	DG	S
JJ	F	1	7,8	B	I	DG	U
CS	F	1	7,8	B	I	DG/CCG	S
CR	F	1	8	U	I	DG	S
BC	F	4	2,4,6	U	D	DG	U
AH	F	4	3,4,6	U	D	DG	S

Type of previous surgery
1 = discoplasty
2 = discectomy
3 = non-specific arthroplasty
4 = alloplastic disc
5 = total joint prosthesis
6 = alloplastic removal
7 = condylectomy
8 = costochondral graft

Reconstructive protocol
I   = immediate
D   = delayed

Reconstructive tissue
D   = dermal graft
CCG = costochondral graft

Outcome
S   = successful
U   = unsuccessful
Q   = questionable

under conditions of "severe fibrous ankylosis" would have ultimately demonstrated true ankylosis had they not been operated is, of course, conjectural. True ankylosis was manifested by obliteration of the articulation with exuberant bone on imaging. In certain of these individuals, slight mobility interincisally was due to the innate elasticity of the mandible. There were 18 patients studied in the "severe fibrous restriction" group, and 18 in the true ankylosis group.

All patients were operated under the same protocol regardless of the diagnosis of fibrous or true ankylosis. Those with no previous history of alloplast placement and those previously operated for ankylosis were all treated by lysis and placement of dermal grafts. When loss of bone substance was significant, placement of costochondral grafts was deferred for a minimum of 12 months. Those individuals in either group who had been treated earlier with alloplasts underwent lysis only at the first operation, and placement of autogenous dermal and/or costochondral grafts only 12 months subsequently,

Table 2. Severe fibrous restriction

Patient	Sex	Number of previous surgeries	Type of previous surgeries	Uni/bi lateral	Reconstructive protocol	Tissue	Outcome
MV	F	6	1,2,4,3	B	D	DG/CCG	S
VP	F	2	1,2,4	U	D	DG	S
RB	F	3	2,4,6	B	D	DG	Q
JA	M	4	1,2,4,6	B	D	DG/CCG	Q
NL	F	2	4,6	B	D	DG/CCG	S
JP	M	4	1,3,4,6	U	D	DG	S
GW	F	21	1,3,2,4,6,5	U	D	DG	S
BS	F	4	2,5,8	B	I	DG	S
DF	F	4	2,4,6	B	I	DG	S
VW	F	1	2,4	B	D	DG/CCG	S
HD	F	1	1	U	I	DG	S
MK	F	2	3,1	U	D	DG/CCG	S
LF	F	1	3,1	U	I	DG	S
MH	F	5	1,4,6,5	B	D	DG/CCG	S
LF	F	4	1,4,5,6	U	I	DG	Q
BC	F	4	2,4,6	U	D	DG	Q
EM	F	7	3,2,3,7	B	D	DG/CCG	S

Type of previous surgery
1 = discoplasty
2 = discectomy
3 = non-specific arthroplasty
4 = alloplastic disc
5 = total joint prosthesis
6 = alloplastic removal
7 = condylectomy
8 = costochondral graft

Reconstructive protocol
I   = immediate
D   = delayed

Reconstructive tissue
D   = dermal graft
CCG = costochondral graft

Outcome
S   = successful
U   = unsuccessful
Q   = questionable

though four of the earlier cases were operated as early as nine months subsequent to the lysis surgery.

Results and discussion

The sole criterion for success in this study was objective demonstration of an interincisal opening of at least 30 mm for at least six months, once attained. This was an easy criterion to fulfill, since in all instances except one (JA in the "severe fibrous restriction" group), lack of success with the procedure became evident well within that six-month period. JA developed an exostosis on a costochondral graft, without re-ankylosis but with attendant decrease in range of motion, some two years following placement of the graft, and required resection of the new mass. No other patient operated under either of the protocols with dermal or dermal and rib grafts developed restriction of movement after the six-month period. A qualified success, as noted in six patients, refers to those individuals who demonstrated distinct and consistent improvement in jaw mobility, but one less than 30 mm, and often accompanied by persistent residual discomfort.

Lateral excursions were not evaluated, since, in most cases, they were absent pre-operatively as a result of previous surgeries. When they returned post-operatively in a few patients, they did so in inconsistent fashion to generally insignificant degree. Neither patient symptomatology nor occlusal status were considered in determining the success or failure of these procedures. Indeed, several patients with successful results in terms of mandibular mobility continued to have at least intermittent discomfort up to two years post-operatively. Similarly, failure of attempts at lysis did not necessarily entail increases in symptomatology post-operatively.

Several patients demonstrated significant occlusal imbalances as a result of extirpation of ankylotic or fibro-ankylotic blocks, some of which were corrected by mandibular repositioning at the time the costochondral grafts were placed. Others underwent subsequent independent orthognathic procedures to improve their occlusions.

Ankylosis or fibro-ankylosis occurred more frequently after removal of alloplastic discs or total joint prostheses than it did while these devices were in place. This finding suggests that the intensity of the foreign body reaction is often severe enough while the inciting factor is in place to provoke an exaggerated healing response after it is removed, and, therewith, fibrosis and/or ossification.

The complexity of the surgical histories of most patients ultimately developing immobility of their articulations is evident in this series, and makes it usually impossible to identify a single previous invasive procedure that has accounted for the ankylosis or fibro-ankylosis. Only nine of the 36 patients in this review, however, had undergone intra-articular procedures alone without the placement of alloplasts of any kind.

The tables also indicate that six patients experienced loss of jaw mobility subsequent to costochondral grafting. One of them (BS) had had her graft placed 11 months previously, concomitant with the removal of a total joint prothesis, around the fossa of which an exuberant foreign body reaction was present. Another four of the six patients (KN, RF, JJ, and CS) developed ankylosis within months of costochondral grafting simultaneously with lysis of earlier ankylosis, but without dermal grafting. This lack of soft tissue interposition played a major role, in the author's opinion, in the development of the subsequent re-ankylosis. The sixth of these patients (CR) was a seven-year old treated with a costochondral graft for correction of hemifacial microsomia, and technical imperfections might well have played a role in the development of her ankylosis. Of the six patients, four (KN, RF, CS, and CR) ranged in age from 4-15 years at the time of their unsuccessful costochondral grafting, emphasizing the role of age in the re-ankylosis tendency. The one unsuccessful case in this series of six patients (JJ) was a patient with severe

generalized rheumatoid arthritis who underwent lysis of her temporomandibular joint ankylosis and bilateral costochondral grafting at age 19, then re-ankylosis, then underwent bilateral lysis of the re-ankylosed joints with concomitant
placement of dermal grafts and costochondral grafts at age 29. By this latter
age, the patient's essential disease had affected the entire spine and all limb
joints. Any further thoughts of lysis of the temporomandibular ankylosis were
abandoned.

Several individual patients in this series merit particular discussion. A
44-year old patient (NK) demonstrated a superb increase in jaw mobility
post-operatively but also developed an epidermal cyst in a dermal graft on one
side which destroyed the roof of the articulation and extended into the middle
cranial fossa. Removal of this cyst resulted in severe neurologic deficits for the
patient which only gradually and incompletely resolved. This case has been
reported earlier.[8] A 22-year old patient (PK) first underwent lysis of peri-articular mandibulo-cranial hyperostosis and only later ankylosis of the temporomandibular joint. Her idiopathic ankylotic pattern became increasingly severe
in subsequent years and spread bilaterally. She remains without definite diagnosis and intractable to all subsequent efforts to mobilize the mandible. Two
patients (GW and BC) demonstrated severe but nonossified restrictions in one
joint, and absolute bony union in the other. They are listed, therefore, in both
tables.

None of these patients underwent programmed intensive physical therapy.
This author has never been convinced of the ultimate advantage of these
interventions and, in fact, has witnessed on occasion an exacerbation of
symptoms or deterioration of results because of premature and/or overly
aggressive efforts at rehabilitation. Whether intensive physical therapy would
have improved the fate of three patients in this group who experienced unquali-
fied failures is very doubtful, in the author's opinion.

Though not executed in every patient in this series, it is the author's opinion
that those patients who, on symptomatic grounds, might be candidates for
surgical intervention because of severely restricted range of motion of the
mandible, but who demonstrate no imaging evidence of ankylosis, should first
undergo examination and manipulation under general anesthesia to isolate any
role of emotion or muscle pain in the patient's complaints or clinical presentation. There is little indication to expose those patients who demonstrate anatomically acceptable range of motion under these circumstances to additional
invasive care.

Conclusion

Qualified success in six and abject failure in three of 36 patients operated under
the described protocols for lysis and autogenous reconstruction of post-surgical
temporomandibular joint ankylosis speak to the validity of these approaches.
Experience with this group of patients suggests that the difference between

severe fibrous restriction and true ankylosis is insignificant in terms of need for and type of lysis, that ankylosis is more frequently encountered after removal of alloplasts than while they are still in place, that costochondral grafting without concomitant placement of a dermal interface in patients treated for ankylosis leads to a rather high rate of re-ankylosis, and that programmed physical therapy is not a major factor in determining the ultimate success in this group of patients. The predictability of undesirable sequelae with the use of autogenous tissues and their general manageability remain, after the prime advantage of host acceptance, the major advantages of autogenous tissues over alloplasts in the lysis of temporomandibular joint ankylosis.

References

1   Eriksson L, Westesson PL. Long-term evaluation of meniscectomy of the temporomandibular joint. J Oral Maxillofac Surg 1985; 43:263
2   Henny FA. Surgical treatment of the painful temporomandibular joint. J Am Dent Assoc 1969; 79:171
3   Silver CM. Long-term results of meniscectomy of the temporomandibular joint. J Craniomandibular Pract 1985; 3:47
4   Tolvanen M, Oikarinen VJ, Wolf J. A 30-year follow-up study of temporomandibular joint meniscectomies: a report on five patients. Br J Oral Maxfac Surg 1988; 26:311
5   Peterson LJ. Multicenter evaluation of temporomandibular joint Proplast-Teflon disc implant. Oral Surg Oral Med Oral Pathol 1992; 74:411
6   Yih WY, Merrill RG. Pathology of alloplastic implants in the temporomandibular joint. Oral Maxillofac Surg Clin North Am 1989; 1:415
7   Jasty M, Smith E. Wear particles of total joint replacements and their role in periprothetic osteolysis. Current Opinion in Rheumatology 1992; 4:204
8   MacIntosh RB. The case for autogenous reconstruction of the adult temporomandibular joint. In: Worthington P, Evans JR (ed). Controversies in Oral and Maxillofacial Surgery. Philadelphia: Saunders 1994; 356
9   Thyne GM, Yoon JH, Luyk NH, McMillan MD. Temporalis muscle as a disc replacement in the temporomandibular joint of sheep. J Oral Maxillofac Surg 1992; 50:979
10 Härle F. Chirurgische Behandlung der Kiefergelenkankyloses mit Interposition von dünnen Knorpelscheiben. Fortschr Kiefer Geschichtschir 1978; 23:139
11 Yih MY, Zysset M, Merrill RG. Histologic study of the fate of autogenous auricular cartilage grafts in the human temporomandibular joint. J Oral Maxillofac Surg 1993; 50:964
12 Stewart H, Hann J, DeTomasi D, et al. Histologic fate of dermal grafts following implantation for temporomandibular joint meniscal perforation: a preliminary study. Oral Surg Oral Med Oral Pathol 1986; 62:481
13 Ware WH, Brown GL. Growth centre transplantation to replace mandibular condyles. J Maxillofac Surg 1981; 9:50
14 Wolford L, Cottrell DA, Henry C. Sternolavicular grafts for temporomandibular joint reconstruction. J Oral Maxfac Surg 1994; 52:119

Management of Temporomandibular
Joint Degenerative Diseases
ed. by B. Stegenga & L.G.M. de Bont
© 1996 Birkhäuser Verlag Basel/Switzerland

Management of non-successful treatment outcome

Ralph G. Merrill

Department of Oral and Maxillofacial Surgery, School of Dentistry, Oregon Health Sciences University, Portland, Oregon 97201-3097, USA

Summary: Many patients who fail temporomandibular joint surgery are left with conditions that are more severe than those that prompted the treatment. The rate of success of repeat surgeries decreases with each additional surgery performed. A careful diagnosis after surgical failure is necessary to discover prior incomplete or inappropriate diagnoses, and misdiagnosis. A concerted effort to treat a patient with failed surgery by non-surgical methods is necessary before proceeding with another surgery. The most conservative, individualized surgical approach should be used when repeat surgery is needed.

Introduction

An accurate incidence of surgical failure for the variety of temporomandibular disorders and surgical procedures is difficult to determine. However, estimates for established procedures range from 10 to 20 percent. Although this apparent failure is a reasonable range, each failed case presents a challenging management problem. Many patients who fail temporomandibular joint surgery are left with conditions that are more severe than their pre-operative status.

Non-successful outcome after surgery of the temporomandibular joint became more prevalent in the 1980s. This is attributed to the dramatic increase in the number of surgeries that were performed for osteoarthrosis and internal derangement, and to the use of interpositional alloplastic implants. The reported rate of failure for patients, not including alloplastic implants, is in the range of 10 to 20 percent. The rate of Proplast-Teflon and planned permanent silastic implants will eventually reach total failure. The perception now is that reactions from Proplast-Teflon are more damaging than from silastic. Failure is often time-related. An implant may fail early and not be recognized until tissue breakdown exceeds tolerance. A delay in the emergence of symptoms may alert the patient sometimes several years later. This is a reason for regular follow-up and evaluation over many years.

One generally accepted standard for the indication for surgery of the temporomandibular joint is that pain and mandibular dysfunction have not been resolved by adequate non-surgical methods. The practitioner considering surgery for such a patient is faced with management of a non-successful treatment outcome to begin with. If the patient is then subjected to surgery, an internal derangement or other arthropathy responsible for the symptoms must be present. The surgeon has the responsibility to determine the adequacy of the non-surgical treatment(s) and that the arthropathy is the primary cause of the signs and symptoms of such a magnitude to justify a surgical approach. Furthermore, the surgeon must determine if referral of pain from other structures is producing signs and symptoms. Contributing psychological disturbances and parafunctional habits must be recognized and treated. When all parts of the puzzle support a surgical approach there is a reasonable chance of a successful surgical outcome. Success does not always depend on restoration of normal anatomic relationships. It is not clear that surgery can prevent or cease progression of the degenerative process. It is safe to say that management of failed surgery is often a complex and demanding task.

Aims of surgical treatment

The aims of temporomandibular joint surgery for initial and repeat procedures are to rid the patient of noxious symptoms, to improve masticatory and oral functions, and to avoid complications. A favorable outcome of surgery sustains a level of pain that is of little or no concern to the patient. The improvement in mandibular function depends on the pre-operative condition whether it be hypomobility from closed-lock, ankylosis, or hypermobility. An interincisal opening greater than 35 mm, lateral excursion greater than 4 mm, and protrusion attaining an end-to-end relationship for incising are considered desirable outcomes. The person should be able to masticate a normal or near normal diet. The occlusion of the teeth should be functional and stable.

The expectation of attaining these goals for the patient with multiple operations is not realistic. Improvements in form and function are more attainable than elimination of chronic pain. A tolerable pain level is possible.

Reasons for surgical failure

Pain of the joint and associated muscles is the foremost symptom that causes the patient to return for treatment. Pain is variable but often chronic. Pain with joint noise during mastication, talking, and yawning are frequent symptoms. Muscle contraction headaches occur frequently. Stress and depression, associated bruxism and sleep disturbances occur. Frustration and anger over unmet expectations contribute to the intensity of the symptoms. Hypomobility resulting from articular and/or myogenous restriction is a common sign of failure. A distorted occlusion and adverse skeletal changes can contribute to the persistence of pain and dissatisfaction. Progressive destructive articular changes are often found in the patient with non-successful outcome. Signs and symptoms of temporomandibular disorders are carefully evaluated in a new thorough differential diagnosis, for previous incomplete or inappropriate diagnosis or misdiagnosis are factors in surgical and non-surgical treatment failures.

Not all jaw and facial pain is due to temporomandibular disorders. Referral of pain to the joint area can originate from any structure of the head and neck.

Myofascial pain and muscle contraction headaches are common maladies in this respect. It is a productive person's disorder affecting the hard-working members of our society who are under stress. Myogenous pain can occur independently or in combination with other disorders of the head and neck. It can be an important muscular splinting component of articular pathology, or it can be independent and coexist with an arthropathy.

The effective management of muscle pain entails patient education and stress reduction. There may be a tendency to overtreat. Surgery is not indicated for isolated muscle pain. Non-surgical care should be conservative. Patients who have a combination of intracapsular and muscular problems usually receive active physical therapy, psychological and/or behavioral treatment, occlusal appliance therapy, and other non-surgical adjunctive care. A surgical procedure, if necessary, can fail if the muscular component is not managed pre- and post-operatively.

An important factor in the success or failure of temporomandibular joint surgery is patient selection.[1] If surgery is a therapeutic option, the patient should be able to accurately describe complaints in a realistic manner. Discussion should ensure that the patient has a clear understanding what the surgery can expect to accomplish and what the limitations of surgery are. The patient must be an active and capable partner in the treatment decisions and in post-surgical rehabilitation. The determination of surgical success depends largely on the patient's perceptions. Therefore, pre-surgical discussions to develop realistic expectations is very important. Behavioral and sociological problems can interfere and need to be addressed in the general plan of treatment.

A multiplicity of etiologic factors affect the outcome of surgery. Intrinsic joint trauma from parafunctional habits is very important in this context. An extrinsic trauma can re-injure the joint sufficiently to require a whole round of new treatment, including surgery.

Reconstructive arthroplasty to reposition and repair a dislocated disc may progressively fail over time without injury. The disc may become dislocated or perforated, leading to further osseous destruction. Escalating osteoarthrotic events may lead to failure and repeat surgery.

An asymptomatic osteoarthrotic joint is not a reason for surgery. Treatment of any kind based on positive radiographs alone is to be avoided. The eventual development of osteoarthrosis and crepitus without other symptomatology does not mean failure. However, severe crepitus, mechanical disturbances in the joint during opening and closing, including catching and locking, are factors in failure. The patient's perception of success and failure is a very important consideration. Advanced pathology can be present in an individual who does not experience noxious symptoms or perceived impaired function. The surgical patient may have these findings years after the surgery but be without symptoms. In the patient's mind surgical treatment has been a success.

The surgical procedure in any case must be selected as a rational response to a specific pathologic condition. The incorrect choice of the operative procedure may result in an additional surgical failure. Disc plication, for example, may not be effective in all situations. Disc removal may be too aggressive. Condylotomy may not be appropriate for advanced internal derangements and with arthrofibrosis from failed arthroscopic or open procedures. Alloplastic implants for disc replacement have been abandoned and total prosthetic joint replacement has become controversial.

The proper application of surgical principles is an important factor in the success of surgery. Intra-operative hemorrhage can result in post-operative hematoma formation leading to slower rehabilitation, increased scar tissue, adhesion formation, and an increased possibility of infection. A meticulous soft tissue dissection combined with appropriate retraction must be employed to prevent excessive bleeding and tissue damage. Adequate access to the joint must be provided by the surgical approach, but careful and conservative incisions decrease the risk of adjacent injury to anatomic structures. Neurologic, vascular, otologic, and infectious complications can occur. Their occurrence in an otherwise technically correct procedure will result in an unsuccessful outcome.

Close and careful follow-up may allow the surgeon to intercept early reversible problems. Adjunctive non-surgical treatment begins pre-operatively and must be continued post-operatively. Inadequate or ineffective physical therapy may result in intracapsular fibrosis and capsulitis. Physical therapy administered under the guidance of an experienced and knowledgeable therapist is important. Improper occlusal therapy will result in an unstable occlusion and undesired loading of the joint in the crucial post-operative period. Throughout all phases of care, a multidisciplinary approach with co-operation and communication is highly desirable.

The source of the initial temporomandibular joint dysfunction may result in or contribute significantly to surgical failure. Failure to diagnose the underlying cause or failure to effectively treat a recognized cause can result in an ineffective surgical therapy. A re-operation may provide initial success but may fail later. Persistence of parafunctional, stress related habits, occlusal instability, and recurrence of injury from other sources may result in a return of pain and dysfunction. The failure to recognize other painful conditions that may co-exist with a temporomandibular disorder (e.g., migraine) can lead to unsuccessful treatment. The patient may believe headaches will be eliminated by surgery, but migraine will not be relieved unless specifically addressed by medication or other specific methods.

All treatment methods will result in a certain number of failures. The success of surgery decreases as the number of surgical procedures increase. Therefore, additional surgeries should be approached with caution.[2]

Management

General considerations

Medical and dental insurance carriers and the providers of care are questioning the necessity of temporomandibular joint surgery. Good arguments can be made for tumor and ankylosis surgery. However, in case of surgery for the relief of pain and dysfunction related to osteoarthrosis and internal derangement it is sometimes more difficult to obtain coverage. It becomes even more difficult to convince others of the necessity to treat individuals who have failed previous surgeries. Not only is it technically and clinically difficult to treat the multiple surgical patient, but it becomes increasingly difficult to gain third party coverage for the necessary hospitalization, surgery, and peri-operative care.

Skills and technology for diagnosis and surgery have had a great impact on the incidence of surgery over the last 15 years. The rapid escalation and the number of surgeries done in the early 1980s would naturally increase the volume of failed surgeries if the rate remained at the 10 to 20 percent level, but we need to consider the much higher rate of failure of patients with alloplastic implants. Alloplastic interpositional implants are no longer commercially available but many individuals still have them in place. Many continue to have significant chronic problems, even though implants have been removed. The old saying "a chance to cut is a chance to cure" characterized the attitude of many surgeons in the early 1980s. Now the philosophy is to be conservative and to know how and when to operate.

It becomes a challenge to determine what realistic options of additional treatment will best resolve the signs and symptoms of the individual with failed surgery. A reasonable approach is the most conservative one to accomplish the aims of pain management and restoration of function. This may range from simple supportive care and jaw rest to the very complex management of problematic patients with implant arthropathy. Complex management may require a team approach to treat chronic pain, stress, depression, persistent articular and peri-articular inflammation, and articular destruction with the resulting skeletal and occlusal distortions.

Many patients who have failed surgery will improve with non-surgical management. Some will not respond to this strategy, however. Reasons vary, but those with pain and dysfunction due to major structural and pathological articular changes and those with chronic pain are important considerations. Those with pain and major structural changes interfering with function usually do well with surgery, whereas those with chronic pain may also need to be in a program with a team of clinicians managing complex contributing factors.

There is a great difference between a failed arthroscopic surgical case and a multiply operated joint. The appropriate approach to take when confronted with a failed surgical case is to begin as one would do with a new patient. A complete re-evaluation is undertaken. A thorough history and physical examination, appropriate imaging and consultations are important. Patient education is necessary to help the patient understand where they stand and what their expectations for success may be. A team approach is indicated for the patient with a history of multiple surgeries and chronic pain. The patient's use or abuse of drugs must be evaluated and acted upon. One must be compassionate and understanding, and listen very carefully to the patient.

The prognosis for success will not only depend on an appropriate and well executed surgery but on an effective rehabilitation program. The patients must be aware and understand their joint pathology, muscle disturbances, parafunctional habits, and other etiologic co-factors. They must be involved in stress management and comply with joint rest, diet modification, home care, and the use of appropriate non-addicting drugs. Medical and dental care must include reassurance for the patient and long-term follow-up. Imaging, physical therapy, occlusal appliance therapy, medications, injections into joints and muscles, arthrocentesis, and pain management are all important considerations in long-term management.

Non-surgical treatment modalities are necessary in both the surgical and the non-surgical patient. Load reduction is very important and is dependent on the patient's motivation and compliance. Since rest means reducing joint loading, the diet must be modified and bruxism controlled. The length of time this is recommended is dependent on the individual's response and may require several months. As with other joint disorders in which inflammation and pain are prominent, non-steroidal anti-inflammatory drugs are indicated. Amitriptyline or other tricyclic drugs in low dosage at bedtime is often useful in controlling bruxism. The pharmacologic control of depression and chronic pain is often necessary. Occlusal appliances are best employed in the treatment of muscular symptoms and may help to decompress the joint. Physical therapy is useful to relieve the musculoskeletal pain and to restore muscular function and mobility. Therapy can reduce inflammation and promote repair and regeneration of tissues. Addressing maladaptive habits and behaviours that stress the masticatory system is an important part of treatment. Treatment may require a psychologist and/or psychiatrist. Psychologic testing can aid in determining prognosis of treatment plans. Behavioral therapy is under-utilized due to attitudes of patients and practitioners.

A failing surgical case discovered early in follow-up can be interpreted and treated successfully by non-surgical methods. A failed surgical case may also be salvaged with a conservative arthrocentesis or arthroscopy without escalating into more complex surgical procedures. However, open procedures for failed cases definitely have their place, including simple to complex reconstructions. Surgical care should be conservative and individualized.

Clinical evaluation and radiography are important for making decisions concerning the type of surgical method necessary. Frequently, however, the final decision is made at the time of surgery while keeping in mind the history, signs and symptoms, and clinical and imaging findings. Clinical, radiographic, and operative findings taken independently do not provide sufficient detail of pathology. By taking all factors into consideration, a reasonable judgement can be made.

The staging of internal derangement is a useful aid in making surgical decisions.[3] In early-intermediate internal derangement, the disc can be successfully repaired. In late-intermediate and late stage internal derangement, the disc cannot be satisfactorily repaired. The geometric distortions of the disc become a consideration for the type of procedure to perform. When morphologic changes prevent the attainment of a functional disc-condyle relationship, then disc repair is not indicated. Removal of the disc is then the most logical option.

There are articular and non-articular disorders that must be dealt with in patients that have failed surgery. Articular problems encountered may include adhesions, capsulitis, synovitis, fibrous and bony ankylosis, disc distortions, osteoarthrosis, rheumatoid arthritis, recurrent luxation, and reactions to implants. Muscular disorders of pain, contractures, otologic symptoms, referred pain from lesions from other head and neck areas, parafunctional habits, psychologic disorders, and chronic pain are several of the non-articular problems to consider when managing the patient with a non-successful treatment outcome.

Arthroscopic failure

The long-term prognosis for the failed arthroscopic procedure is usually favorable. An arthrocentesis can be performed initially, which is diagnostic and therapeutic. The repeat surgical approach for failed arthroscopic surgery can be either an arthroscopic procedure or an open procedure of disc repair or discectomy. When the disc is removed because of advanced pathology it is rarely necessary to use an autogenous graft. The literature and experience of many surgeons is supportive of discectomy without the interposition of a replacement.[4]

The conservative approach rather than escalation is desirable for the patient with a non-successful treatment outcome. The conservative procedure of arthroscopic lysis and lavage is a reasonable option. The decision to re-operate a joint requires re-evaluation of both the existing pathology as well as a re-assessment of why previous attempts have failed. Management problems often escalate with each additional surgery and the patient may well be on the road to fibrosis, articular degeneration, chronic pain and dysfunction. The previously operated joint is less resistant to repeat injury than the unoperated joint.

Arthroscopic surgical techniques provide options for less aggressive, less invasive management of the failed or failing case. Arthroscopic surgery can provide therapeutic relief for painful hypomobility due to adhesions. A lysis and lavage can eliminate adhesions and allow mobilization of the joint. Not all patients will improve with arthroscopic surgery but the incidence of worsening of a patient's condition is very small. Arthrotomy in the best of conditions will result in greater bleeding and scar formation. Joints which have undergone discectomy, disc repair, and autogenous reconstruction are all potential candidates for an arthroscopic approach. However, patients with extensive fibrous ankylosis and those with alloplastic implants will require an open surgical revision.

Immediate post-operative home exercises and physical therapy can be employed as there are no suture lines to disrupt. The surgical access is less traumatic and the patient will have less pain and consequently will be able to exercise their jaw early. As with any surgical procedure, there is a potential for articular scar tissue formation. Accordingly, the patient's commitment and participation in the rehabilitation process is essential. The patient must have a good understanding of the mechanism which led to the poor result from earlier surgical attempts, and must be an active partner in preventing the same course of events to occur again.

Arthrotomy failure

Arthroscopic surgical revision is usually not effective in the presence of advanced pathology. Arthrotomy procedures become necessary. This is decided at the time of diagnostic arthroscopy or in lieu of arthroscopy. An open procedure to remove the pathology with the possible use of an interposition of autogenous tissue is usually more effective than arthroscopic procedures in this situation. Fibrous and bony ankylosis, condylar necrosis, tumors, and destructive implant arthropathy are conditions that require an open approach.

The decision to use or not to use an autogenous tissue graft is a controversial subject. A growing number of surgeons prefer not to use a graft or implant, and depend on physical therapy and biologic adaptation of articular tissues. Alloplastic material for articular reconstruction is not recommended due to the probability of displacement, fragmentation, foreign body granuloma formation, regional adenopathy, erosion of articular bone, condylar necrosis, ankylosis, infection, chronic foreign body reaction, apertognathia, retrognathia, and chronic pain. Autogenous tissues used for interposition include temporalis fascia, myofascial temporalis flaps, conchal cartilage, dermis, fascia, and, for condylar reconstruction, the costochondral graft.

The re-operated joint with a small intra-articular gap and minimal articular destruction with fibrous tissue covering bone can be successfully treated by an open arthrolysis followed by intensive physical therapy and joint mobilization. Articular fusion may recur and it is not yet established if a thin temporalis flap or conchal cartilage graft will be more reliable in the prevention of ankylosis. Conchal cartilage can be used to repair fossa defects or severe thinning of temporal bone. Nearly complete or complete loss of the condyle and shortening of the mandibular ramus may require reconstruction with a costochondral graft and possibly a fossa lining of either temporalis, conchal cartilage, or dermis. An alternative is total joint reconstruction using metal articulating against plastic. However, in view of the present state of the art and the desirability of biologic surgery, autogenous reconstruction is preferred. The safety and efficacy of prosthetic total joint replacement is yet to be determined.

Another option in the patient with a large articular defect after revision surgery is not to use tissue for reconstruction, and to aid occlusal and skeletal adaptation with the prolonged use of maxillo-mandibular guiding elastics and physical therapy.[5] Mandibular exercises are frequent with periodic removal of elastics each day.

The aims of treatment are to improve jaw function and to reduce pain to tolerable levels. Expectation of a complete cure is not realistic. The patient who has failed multiple non-surgical and surgical procedures often suffers with chronic pain, psychological disturbance, malocclusion, jaw deformity, muscle contractures, and significant joint destruction. A team approach is usually necessary for the successful management of this difficult category of patients. Chronic pain management, counseling, orthodontics, orthognathic surgery, physical therapy, and restorative occlusal management are important considerations in addition to the technically difficult reconstructive joint procedures that may be necessary.

Disc repair and discectomy failure

When disc repair and discectomy procedures fail, the treatment approach involves a complete re-assessment, home care, and non-surgical care. If surgery then becomes necessary, the preferred surgery is arthroscopy. Diagnostic arthroscopy can reveal adhesiveness, chondromalacia, synovitis, and other pathology that may contribute to or cause the patient's problem. Arthrofibrosis is the most common finding in both discectomy and repair cases and can be corrected by arthroscopic lysis to regain function and reduce symptoms. The presence of advanced disc pathology in the failed disc repair case usually means disc removal. The articular bearing surfaces most often have a fibrous tissue cover and, if not disturbed, an autogenous interpositional graft is not necessary. The judicious use of an autogenous graft is an option in the presence of articular bony degeneration in both failed disc repair and removal cases. The necessity of using any type of interpositional graft remains controversial. An aggressive physical therapy rehabilitation program is necessary in any case after repeat surgery involving arthrofibrosis.

Alloplast failure

Alloplastic materials used for temporomandibular joint disc replacement and reconstruction are not all equal. Although they are different, fragmentation occurs with any implant. The main implants used in the early 1980s are silastic, silastic with dacron reinforcement, and Proplast-Teflon. Total prosthetic joints consisted of different combinations of metal alloys, acrylic, and high molecular weight polyethylene. The long-term prognosis including the elimination of pain and regaining normal jaw function for most patients with Proplast-Teflon implants is poor. Prognosis is guarded for silastic. Patient with these implants develop pain, restriction of opening, occlusal-skeletal changes, and many other clinical signs and symptoms. These symptoms may develop months to years after the initial implant surgery. Management of the failures can be simple implant removal or complex removal, debridement, and reconstruction. Foreign body reactions in articular and peri-articular tissues can be identified years after removal of an implant. This may contribute to an increase in failures when for reconstruction autogenous tissues are used.[6]

The American Association of Oral and Maxillofacial Surgeons convened a 22 participant workshop on temporomandibular joint implant surgery.[7] Each participant had expertise in the management of temporomandibular joint disorders and in addition had critically reviewed hundreds of related scientific articles supplied to them prior to the workshop. The charges of the participants were to develop a consensus concerning the use of interpositional and reconstructive materials in the temporomandibular joint and to develop a consensus concerning the management of patients in whom temporomandibular joint implants had been placed and who are either symptomatic or asymptomatic at the time of presentation.

There were several pertinent general recommendations by the workshop:

- The use of Proplast-Teflon interpositional implants should be discontinued since it is an inappropriate material for this purpose.
- The permanent placement of silastic as an interpositional material in the temporomandibular joint should no longer be done, except when used to prevent recurrence of ankylosis. There was a diversity of opinion concerning the use of planned temporary silastic following discectomy. Silastic was withdrawn from the market by the manufacturer.
- Alloplastic total joint replacement is an option in patients with extensive temporomandibular joint disease. However, because the long-term outcome of currently available total joints has not yet been determined, prosthetic total joints should be considered only when their safety and efficacy have been established.
- Discectomy without replacement accompanied by physical therapy is an acceptable procedure when there are minimal bony changes. However, in patients with more extensive bony change, disc replacement may be necessary with autogenous tissue.
- A costochondral graft is the currently preferred material for condylar replacement when autogenous tissue is used. Autogenous tissue is also appropriate for disc and fossa repair and replacement for use as an interpositional material to prevent re-ankylosis and for augmentation of the articular eminence.

Recommendations for the management of patients who have received alloplastic temporomandibular joint implants were organized into four categories, depending on their clinical and imaging status at the time of presentation:

Category I: the patient is asymptomatic and has no changes on imaging.
Category II: the patient is asymptomatic, but has imaging changes.
Category III: the patient is symptomatic without imaging changes.
Category IV: the patient is symptomatic with imaging changes.

Failed Proplast-Teflon
For category I patients it is recommended to remove the implant and affected soft tissues. The patient should be followed post-operatively with magnetic resonance imaging and computerized tomography yearly for at least two years, then discontinued when asymptomatic and without evidence of progressive imaging changes. If symptoms and imaging changes develop, removal of residual soft tissue reaction may be indicated. The management of categories II, III and IV are basically the same. It is recommended to remove the implant along with the affected soft tissues and followed post-operatively with magnetic resonance imaging and computerized tomography yearly for five years, and then discontinued if asymptomatic and stable on imaging. Re-operation and further debridement may be necessary if symptoms develop or recur. If there are no imaging changes present, replacement after implant removal may not be necessary. If bony changes are present, reconstruction, if required, may be immediate or delayed using autogenous tissue or possibly a total joint prosthesis for which the safety and efficacy have been established.

If the patient refuses implant removal, it is recommended to follow the patient every six months with clinical examination and magnetic resonance imaging indefinitely. At removal, if it is deemed necessary to use a replacement, autogenous tissue is recommended. If there is a large perforation into the middle cranial fossa, repair with an autogenous graft is indicated.

It was the experience of several participants of the workshop that reactive tissue and bone degeneration are usually greater than shown by radiographic imaging.

Prosthetic total joint failure
For the category I patient it is recommended to evaluate yearly by clinical examination and radiographic imaging.

The category II patient should have baseline radiographic imaging, then repeated at six months to see if the condition is stable or progressive. If stable, the patient should be followed at yearly intervals. If changes are progressive, the total joint prosthesis should be removed and replaced with a costochondral graft, or possibly by another total joint prosthesis for which safety and efficacy have been established. The patient should be evaluated yearly by clinical examination and radiographic imaging.

The category III patient should be evaluated clinically and radiographically to rule out other causes of symptoms. If the condition is caused by implant failure and foreign body reaction, removal of the total joint and debridement of the area and replacement with a costochondral graft or another joint prosthesis is indicated. Yearly evaluation by clinical examination and radiographic imaging is recommended.

In the category IV patient the total joint should be removed with debridement of the area and replacement with a costochondral graft or another total joint prosthesis. Yearly clinical and radiographic evaluation is recommended for follow-up.

Silastic failure

The consensus was that silastic is in general less damaging to the joint than Proplast-Teflon. However, close follow-up and a strong inclination for removal was the predominant opinion of the workshop participants.

In category I, it was advised that the patient be counseled about the benefits of retaining or removing the implants. If the patient chooses to retain the implant, follow-up with computerized tomography or radiography yearly for at least two years is recommended. If the condition remains stable, the patient should be advised of the need for periodic follow-up examinations.

The patient in category II should be similarly advised as category I patients. If the patient chooses to retain the implant, computerized tomography or radiography should be done at six months to determined if imaging changes are progressing. If changes are progressive then the implant should be removed; if the previously observed changes are stable, repeat computerized tomography or radiography should be advised yearly for at least two years. If the condition continues to remain stable, the patient should be advised of the need for periodic follow-up examinations.

The category III patient should be advised of the risks and benefits of retaining or removing the implant. If the patient chooses to retain the implant, the patient should be provided supportive care and follow-up with computerized tomography or radiography at six months. If the symptoms persist at six months, the implants should be removed. If the patient becomes asymptomatic and chooses to retain the implant, it is recommended to repeat computerized tomography or radiography at six months and then yearly for at least two years. If the condition remains stable, the patient should be advised of the need for periodic follow-up examination.

The category IV patient should be advised of risks and benefits. If imaging changes are slight, supportive care should be provided and follow-up should be done with computerized tomography or radiography at six months. If imaging changes are progressive the patient is advised to have the implant removed, and if the imaging changes remain stable, imaging at six months and then yearly for at least two years is advised. If the condition continues to remain stable, the patient is advised of the need for periodic follow-up examination. If imaging changes are moderate to severe, the patient should be advised to have the implant removed, but if the patient chooses to retain the implant, supportive care should be provided and follow-up computerized tomography or radiography should be done at six months. If at six months imaging changes are progressive and symptoms persist, the patient should be advised to have the implant removed. If the patient becomes asymptomatic and chooses to retain the implant, repeat computerized tomography or radiography and clinical examination should be done at six months and then yearly for at least two years. If the condition remains stable, the patient should be advised of the need for periodic follow-up examinations.

If the patient elects to have the implant removed in any of the categories, the option to not replace or to replace the implant with autogenous tissue are both acceptable methods. There is evidence clinically and radiographically of fragmentation, displacement, and tears in silastic implants occurring many years after they were placed. Therefore, long-term follow-up examinations indefinitely are prudent.

Summary and conclusions

Surgery is a method of managing failed non-surgical treatments when impaired function and pain are due to an arthropathy. The rate of success for an initial surgery is remarkably 80 to 90 percent. Many patients who fail temporo-mandibular joint surgery are left with conditions that are more severe than their pre-operative status. The rate of success of repeat surgeries decreases with each additional surgery performed.

A careful diagnosis after surgical failure is necessary to discover prior incomplete and inappropriate diagnoses, and misdiagnosis. Contributing behavioral disturbances, parafunctional habits, sources of referred pain (e.g., myofascial pain), and co-existing painful conditions such as migraine must be identified and managed.

A concerted effort to treat a patient with failed surgery by non-surgical methods is necessary before proceeding with another surgery. The most conservative, individualized surgical approach should be used when repeat surgery is needed. An arthroscopic procedure is used when possible. If arthroscopy is not appropriate, arthrotomy techniques of disc preservation or disc removal (preferably without replacement) are indicated. The eventual failure of all alloplastic reconstructions of the disc and joint is expected.

Treatment can be complex, often requiring team management and surgery including simple implant removal to complex debridement and reconstruction with autogenous tissue. A costochondral graft for replacement of a condyle is preferred over an alloplastic joint replacement until safety and efficacy of a total joint prosthesis is proven.

References

1 Sanders B, Buoncristiani RD. Temporomandibular joint arthrotomy, management of failed cases. Oral Maxillofac Surg Clin North Am 1989; 2:443
2 Bradrick JP, Indresano AT. Failure rate of repetitive temporomandibular joint procedures. J Oral Maxillofac Surg 1992; 50:145
3 Bronstein SL. Guidelines for temporomandibular joint arthroscopy. In: Thomas M, Bronstein SL. Arthroscopy of the temporomandibular joint. Philadelphia: Saunders, 1991; 229
4 Eriksson L, Westesson PL. Long-term evaluation of meniscectomy of the temporomandibular joint. J Oral Maxillofac Surg 1985; 43:263
5 Swift JQ. Salvage of the TMJ by removing Proplast implant and thorough debridement without joint replacement. J Oral Maxillofac Surg 1994; 52:18
6 Henry HH, Wolford LM. Treatment outcomes for temporomandibular joint reconstruction after Proplast-Teflon implant failure. J Oral Maxillofac Surg 1993; 51:352
7 American Association of Maxillofacial Surgeons Special Committee on TMJ implants. Recommendations for management of patients with TMJ implants. J Oral Maxillofac Surg 1993; 51:1164

Synthesis

Management of Temporomandibular
Joint Degenerative Diseases
ed. by B. Stegenga & L.G.M. de Bont
© 1996 Birkhäuser Verlag Basel/Switzerland

Discussion of controversial statements

John F. Helfrick

Department of Oral and Maxillofacial Surgery, University of Texas at Houston, Health Science Center, Dental Branch, Houston, Texas 77030, USA

Introduction

As a synthesis, seven controversial statements have been discussed at the International TMJ Congress by an expert panel, consisting of Drs. Alastair Goss (Australia), Lars Eriksson (Sweden), and Jeffrey Okeson (USA), and by conference participants.

Statement 1

The temporomandibular joint is a synovial joint like all others and it is becoming obvious that enzymatic pathways are involved in cartilage matrix degradation. In addition, temporomandibular joint osteoarthrosis may cause disc displacement.

Dr. Alastair Goss stated that he agreed with this statement and urged that other members of the dental profession be made aware of the importance of understanding the biologic basis for temporomandibular joint osteoarthrosis. He stated that the temporomandibular joint is not a "different" joint from other joints within the body and that in order to fully understand the pathophysiology of osteoarthrosis, we must become biochemists as well as anatomists and physiologists.

Dr. Lars Eriksson also agreed with this statement and made a plea for the consideration of discectomy as a method for the management of advanced disc disease and osteoarthrosis. In a recent review of the literature he did not find any paper which showed that any biological or alloplastic material used to replace the disc is superior to merely performing a discectomy without replacement. He pointed out that, although the joints do not appear healthy radiographically and may have joint crepitus, the patients state that they feel better and are noted to have a good range of motion following discectomy without replacement.

These findings were challenged by Dr. Robert MacIntosh (USA) who stated that he had reviewed his personal experience while on the faculty at Henry Ford Hospital and noted that Dr. Fred Henny, who had originally advocated the discectomy procedure, later abandoned the operation because of an excessively high morbidity rate noted in these patients. Dr. MacIntosh expressed concern with his follow-up of these patients where four had severe/profound ankylosis. He noted that many of the articles published on this subject failed to identify post-surgical range of motion and the presence or absence of malocclusions.

Dr. Eriksson then countered that malocclusion had not been a finding in their patients. Dr. Anders Holmlund (Sweden) stated that his success rates were similar to those of Eriksson in a prospective study where an 85% long term success rate was noted with the discectomy procedure. He and Dr. MacIntosh agreed that the differences may be in patient selection and that Dr. MacIntosh, who admitted that he does not perform the discectomy procedure, may be seeing only the problems of other surgeons.

Statement 2

Surgical therapy should be considered only after reasonable non-surgical efforts have failed and the patient's quality of life is being significantly affected.

Dr. Jeffrey Okeson (USA) made a plea for consideration of surgery only after non-surgical methods of management had been unsuccessful. He stressed the importance of the psychological evaluation of the chronic pain patient and pointed out that surgery in some of these patients may in fact compound the "psychological axis" of these patients secondary to their pre-existing so-cial/psychological problems. He noted that we should be very careful of patients with somatoform complaints, e.g. leg pain and back pain, and that a joint operation probably won't help and may, in fact, compound the problems of these patients. If non-surgical therapy is failing you must be sure that you are dealing with intracapsular pain. The patient may be having referred cervical pain and Dr. Okeson recommended a diagnostic auriculotemporal nerve block as a method of obtaining a differential diagnosis. If the block is unsuccessful in eliminating the pain, the practitioner should look for another diagnosis and another source for the patient's pain. Failure of otherwise excellent therapeutic modalities to resolve the pain may be secondary to a diagnostic failure. He urged that surgeons not operate merely to manage pain and that, prior to proceeding with surgery, a cause for the pain must be identified. He made the important point that neuropathic pain concepts have changed and that we now understand that many of the patients with chronic pain have a central, rather than peripheral (temporomandibular joint) problem. Performing operations on the temporomandibular joint in these patients is destined to failure.

Dr. Geert Boering (The Netherlands) followed this statement with a caution for surgeons to not operate on the basis of a "bad X-ray". He pointed out that the disease may very well have "burned out" and that you are merely seeing the residual results of the remodeling process.

Dr. Michael Koslin (USA) cautioned that long-term non-invasive/non-surgical therapy is also not indicated, and that many temporomandibular joint problems are best treated when they are in their acute phase. He urged for the consideration of arthrocentesis in the acute patient versus long-term non-surgical therapy.

Dr. Dorrit Nitzan (Israel) stressed that in acute closed-lock, physical therapy is contra-indicated. She stated that aggressive physical therapy in these patients will, in fact, cause progression of the disease, i.e., further disc displacement. She agreed with Dr. Koslin for consideration of arthrocentesis in these acute closed-lock cases.

Statement 3

Modified condylotomy for management of early internal derangement results in increased joint space, a changed condylar position, and in joint healing.

Dr. Goss spoke in opposition to condylotomy for the management of internal derangement of the temporomandibular joint. He stated "I have never done one and do not believe in it!". He noted that the work performed by Sir Terrence Ward and Professor Peter Banks had been quoted by Dr. Samuel McKenna (USA) in his presentation on the use of the condylotomy procedure for the management of internal derangements. Dr. Goss noted that the work by Drs. Ward and Banks included a very heterogenous group of patients and that many had neuromuscular problems rather than internal derangement of the temporo-mandibular joint. Therefore, he stressed that reference to this paper does not support Dr. McKenna's contention that the condylotomy procedure is effective.

Dr. McKenna was just as strong in his response and stated "I have no doubts about the efficacy of this procedure in the treatment of patients with early internal derangement". He stated that the best results are achieved in patients with Wilkes' stage II and stage III internal derangements.

Dr. Okeson requested that surgeons consider the use of an anterior reposi-tioning splint and, if the effects are good, he recommended continued use of the orthotic in an attempt to avoid surgery. Dr. McKenna agreed with the early use of splints. However, he stated that splints should not be used for a long period of time since this will result in irreversible disc changes and a dental malocclusion. He stated that "a trial of a repositioning splint is certainly acceptable but should be discontinued prior to the creation of a non-reducing disc". Dr. Okeson asked what the condyle to disc relationship is following the condylotomy procedure. Dr. McKenna answered by stating that at ten years 60% of the discs are in normal position as noted both on sagittal and coronal magnetic resonance imaging examinations.

Dr. Joseph McCain (USA) expressed concern with the condylotomy proce-dure, which causes "condylar sag and resultant bite abnormalities". He has noted in patients in which this procedure has been used for the correction of Class III mandibular deformities, that many of them had posterior premature contacts after the surgery. Dr. McKenna noted that there is a difference between treating a case of mandibular prognathism with a condylotomy procedure and treating a patient who has otherwise normal/habitual occlusion with this operation for the management of internal joint derangement. In the paper in which he and Drs. Hall and Nickerson reported on 400 patients, there was a 1-2% incidence of malocclusion, and he believed that this was certainly acceptable.

Dr. Robert Walker (USA) supported Dr. McKenna's comments and stated that it is "the easiest operation I do". He noted that he merely creates what are essentially bilateral subcondylar fractures, places the patient into intermaxillary fixation for three days, and then places the patient into training elastics until his (her) occlusion is repeatable. He believes that this approach gives very excellent and predictable results for the management of early temporomandibular joint internal derangement.

Statement 4

Because results of temporomandibular joint arthroscopic lysis and lavage in Wilkes' stage III or higher seem to be better than those reported after temporomandibular joint disc repair procedures, there is no rationale for disc repair procedures.

Dr. Eriksson is not sure that this statement is correct and is not aware of any randomized studies which compare the results of these two techniques. Dr. Goss also disagreed with the statement and would discourage the acceptance of this concept until more randomized studies have been published.

Dr. Okeson pointed out that the post-operative results reported in most scientific articles following different surgical procedures are the same ... 80% of the patients get better. He went on to state that we must get better at defining our patient populations and relating the diagnoses to a more definitive definition of the surgical procedure and outcome criteria. In a recent study from a group in Montreal, patients who wore sham appliances versus the standard orthotic, improved at the same rate (i.e., 80% got better), and Dr. Okeson used this paper to point out the importance of the placebo effect. However, he also stated that the placebo effect is a powerful modality that should not be ignored and can be utilized effectively to manage patients.

Dr. Robert Schwartz (USA) stated that the philosophy of the surgeon is extremely important in the selection of the operation. Some surgeons philosophically believe that it is critical to restore anatomical form and function to the joint in order to prevent progression of the disorder. However, there are others who believe that by doing the least invasive procedure, a patient will experience the best results in the long-term as these procedures allow the patient to adapt. Dr. Schwartz's desire is to do the least invasive procedure required in order to restore function and to decrease pain. This will ultimately give the patient the best results.

Dr. McCain agreed and stated that his approach is to, initially, perform arthrocentesis under local anesthesia, and if this is not effective in eliminating the closed-lock he would then move ahead immediately with arthroscopy performed under local anesthesia in the office.

Dr. Mark Piper (USA) made the point that most of the publications show that arthroscopy is effective only in early cases of internal derangement. He also stressed that we should not overlook the importance of medial versus lateral pole disc displacement. His experience is that management of lateral pole displacement of the disc does not require any invasive approach and that these problems should be treated non-surgically.

Dr. William McCarty (USA) stated that in Wilkes' stage III, IV and V, the disc is not amenable to repair. His approach is to perform a discectomy for this group of patients and he does not use an interpositional material. He is a strong proponent of arthrocentesis in virgin joints and believes that it is very "cost effective". Because the current literature shows high success rates in early closed-lock cases with arthrocentesis, and since this approach cost 10% that of arthroscopy, he will initially perform arthrocentesis and if this fails he will proceed to arthroscopy.

Statement 5

Temporomandibular joint arthrocentesis seems to have the potential to claim a similar percentage of success as obtained with arthroscopic lysis and lavage in temporomandibular joint internal derangement and degenerative diseases.

When asked whether she ever performs arthroscopy, Dr. Dorrit Nitzan (Israel) responded that in her studies she found the same success between arthrocentesis and arthroscopic lysis and lavage. In addition, she has noted an increased mouth opening in the arthrocentesis patients and attributes this to possible scar tissue formed as a result of arthroscopy; therefore, she limits the management of early internal derangement to the arthrocentesis procedure.

Dr. Nitzan also related her results of arthrocentesis for the management of osteoarthrosis in 15 patients. She found in her study that 10 of the patients responded very well to arthrocentesis and did not require any additional therapy. However, five patients showed no improvement and required an open joint procedure. She concluded, therefore, that even in cases of advanced degenerative disease, arthrocentesis should be considered before moving to open joint surgery. She also stated that Wilkes' stage I and II patients with or without pain benefit from arthrocentesis. She stated that "patients should not be told that they have to wait until they have closed-lock before they qualify for arthrocentesis".

Dr. Frank Dolwick (USA) stated that we should be cautious about recommending arthrocentesis for Wilkes' stage III patients as the research results from this group are inconclusive. He pointed out that Dr. Nitzan's patients

primarily comprise those with an "anchored disc" and sudden restricted opening. He stated that this is the group that obtains the best results from arthrocentesis. Patients with a history of intermittent clicking or locking over a long
period of time have not done as well as those with sudden acute locking. Dr.
Dolwick recommended arthrocentesis under local anesthesia, and, as Dr.
McCain had previously suggested, he would evaluate the patient's response
and move directly to arthroscopic lysis and lavage if the closed-lock did not
resolve.

Dr. Lambert de Bont (The Netherlands) stressed that we need randomized
studies so that Wilkes' stage III patients, with controls, are scientifically
studied. He went on to state that objective studies are imperative and that we
should avoid the publication of reports which stress the subjective responses
of patients to various surgical procedures.

Statement 6

Avascular necrosis of the mandibular condyle is uncommon.

Dr. Eriksson commented that he and Dr. Per-Lennart Westesson have biopsied
35 condylar heads and "two or three could be classified as having avascular
necrosis" according to a pathologist in Rochester, New York. He also stated
"we have seen it but we do not know the significance".

Dr. Goss also stated that he has seen very few cases that could be described
as avascular necrosis and has assumed that this is a rare condition.

Dr. Okeson stated that he has seen only three or four patients where there
has been significant condylar head resorption in his many years of treating
temporomandibular joint patients and believes that this must be a very uncommon condition.

Dr. Piper stated that he sees avascular necrosis patients because, although
these are very uncommon cases, they are referred to him after others have made
the diagnosis radiographically.

Dr. Walker stated that avascular necrosis is very uncommon. He has seen
two cases in 40 years of practice and urged that these patients be treated
non-surgically with the application of arch bars and the use of interarch elastics.
Within six months these patients have a new articulation formed and his patients
have done very well without surgical management. He has reviewed his cases
involving benign condylar tumors which resulted in condylar head resection
without replacement. Arch bars and intermaxillary fixation with elastics were
used with predictable occlusal and functional results. He urged the attendees
to consider very conservative management of this very uncommon avascular
necrosis problem. Dr. Walker also stated that we should "... get rid of the term
'conservative'. Wrong treatment is never conservative." The proper terms are
either surgical or non-surgical treatment.

Dr. Boering has reviewed his cases and had not found many cases which could be considered avascular necrosis. However, he is intrigued by the cases of the "juvenile form of osteoarthrosis" which he stated look very much like avascular necrosis. He stated, however, that he has not been able to prove that the resorptive process seen in younger patients is, in fact, avascular necrosis.

Statement 7

Physical therapy is not a major factor in the efficacy of surgical treatment.

Dr. Goss stated that this would be a correct statement if we would eliminate the word "not". He stated that the best thing that he has ever done in the management of his temporomandibular joint patients is to develop a good working relationship with a physical therapist.

Dr. Nitzan stressed the importance of motion in the joint. She referred to research that shows that motion decreases joint pressure and improves blood and fluid flow within the joint. Dr. Walker also stressed the importance of physical therapy in the management of temporomandibular disorders.

Dr. Helfrick pointed out that there is no standardization to physical therapy protocols and that well-controlled clinical research projects are needed to identify the best methods of physical therapy for temporomandibular joint patients. Dr. MacIntosh also recommended prospective studies to evaluate the effects of physical therapy over time to see how patients who receive standardized physical therapy progress versus those who receive no physical therapy following temporomandibular joint procedures.

Conclusion

The consensus following the panel discussion was that, although tremendous progress is being made, there is still a great deal to be learned about the pathophysiology of the temporomandibular joint. Basic research should provide a biologic basis for proper management of disorders affecting the joint. All were in agreement that prospective randomized studies are subsequently needed to evaluate treatment outcome. This would provide the best opportunity for solving the many questions concerning this very complex anatomical structure.

Subject index

234

236

Lightning Source UK Ltd.
Milton Keynes UK
UKHW020952090219

336892UK00003B/180/P